Cullen's Egg Bottle

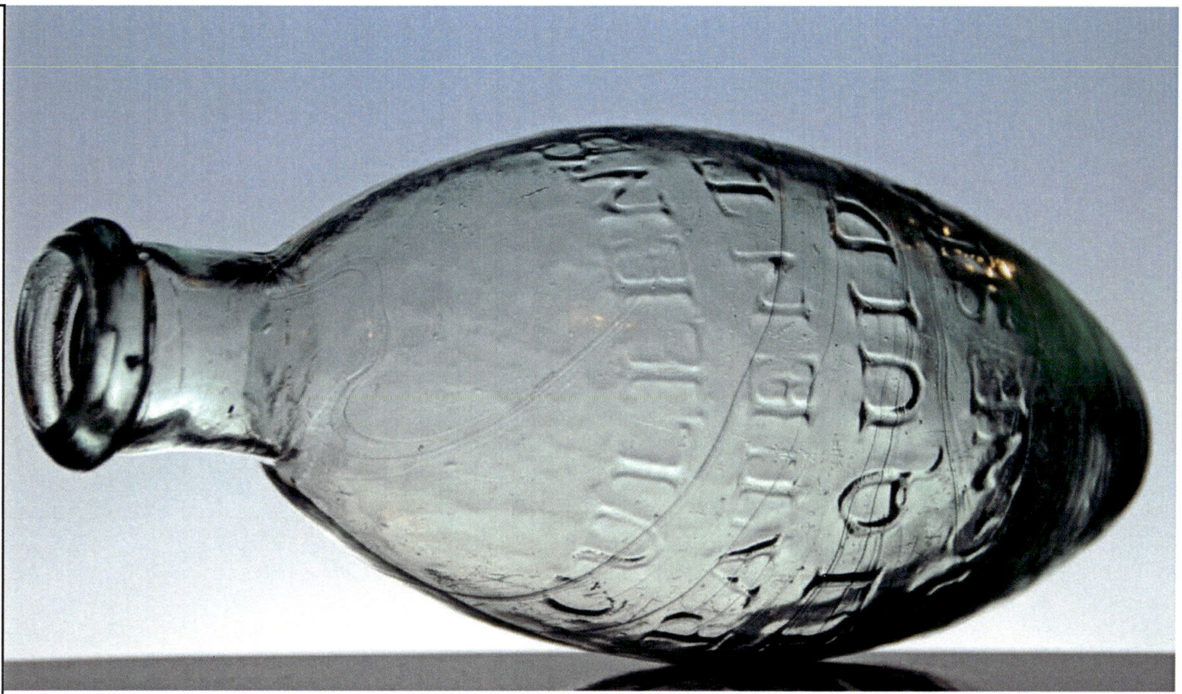

Through Historical Illumination, A United States Treasure Is Discovered as We Follow The Trail to the Tale

Lost in Time,
But for A Lone Artifact
Showing Us
How to Remember

This is a wonderful story about an American archeological mystery solved by following a series of historical clues.

Abstract

Come, walk with the author as he discovers the earliest known US embossed artificial mineral water bottle and its wonderful tale of US firsts – a "*national treasure*" that rewrites history in the early US period (1800-1840). Enjoy the thrill and excitement of touching history through John Cullen's wonderful accomplishments. Weaving an anecdotal first person narration, the author stresses a scientific approach to historical archaeology. The view is from Philadelphia as Cullen emerges in 1818 at 22 years of age, then moves forward and backward chronologically - exploring *"Full Historic"* interactions across regions and continents as it applies to our tale. Cultural and environmental transitions sweep in all directions that can hardly be imagined by just considering the artifact itself, "*Cullen's egg bottle*". Following a trail of newly discovered archaeological evidence and associated "original source documents" (OSD), an entirely new historical perspective will emerge, illuminating both professionals and amateurs alike.

Supplementary Appendix material, (OSD), explores the origins and roots of the US artificial mineral and soda water industry. Most of the Appendix is of first impression, never before known or understood. This plenary supplement will be referenced in the author's 9 volume series and should be viewed as a prerequisite to several of these volumes. Each succeeding volume will be released individually at a future date.

Internet keys: John Cullen M.D.; Philadelphia Pa.; Paris, France; Richmond Va.; Napoleon Bonaparte; Thomas Jefferson; John Syng Dorsey; Egg Bottles; Antique Bottles; Archaeology; Privy / Privies; University of Pennsylvania; Virginia Commonwealth University; VCU; MCV; Medical College of Virginia; Hampden–Sydney College; Thomas W. Dyott; Charlotte Howard Cullen; John Redmond Coxe M.D.; slavery; Jacob Schweppe; Elias Durand; James S. Ewing; Joseph Hawkins; Abraham H. Cohen; Liquid Magnesia; Mineral Water; Soda Water; Seltzer Water; soda fountain; X patents; Hydrant; pontil; Philadelphia Medical Museum; freeze valves; remote controlled valves; hydraulic valves; water hydrants; torpedo bottles; pontilled; historical archaeology; provenience; full history; US Early period history; OSD; Eugene Roussel; American Philosophical Society; Magellanic Premium Award; flavored mineral water; Henry G. Douglass; pottery bottles; John Syng Dorsey Cullen M.D.; John M. Matthews; reconstructed patents; US patents; X patents; John Cotter; American cultural anthropology; torpedo bottles; England; Ireland; Dublin; Schweppe & Co.; UK;

Tales Derived
from Artifact Context
and Historical Records

In America's Pre-Civil War Past
Volume 1

Cullen's Egg Bottle

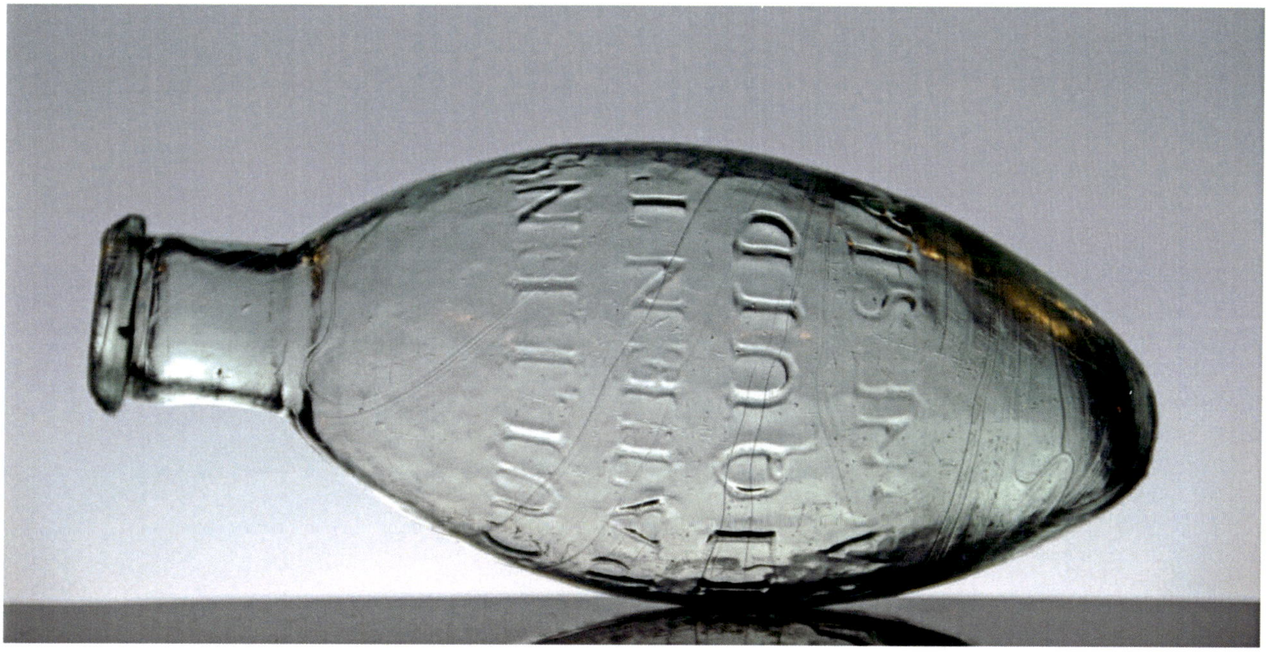

Philo Gideon

An Academic Series
Referenced solely by Original Source Documents

Printed and bound in the United States of America

PhiloGideon@Yahoo.Com

First printing - August 2008

ISBN: 978-0-9819157-0-8

10987654321

Hidden Tales

Dedication

Discovery of this wonderful history would not have been possible without the tremendous sacrifices of my wife Jan. With love, understanding, and patience, she has supported my adventures and dreams over a lifetime. I hope in some small measure this will justify her faith in me.

Illustrations

Epigraph

Archaeology is for everyone, everywhere, and surrounds all of us in our daily lives. Competent independent archaeologists and amateurs will continue to flourish making significant contributions of first impression.

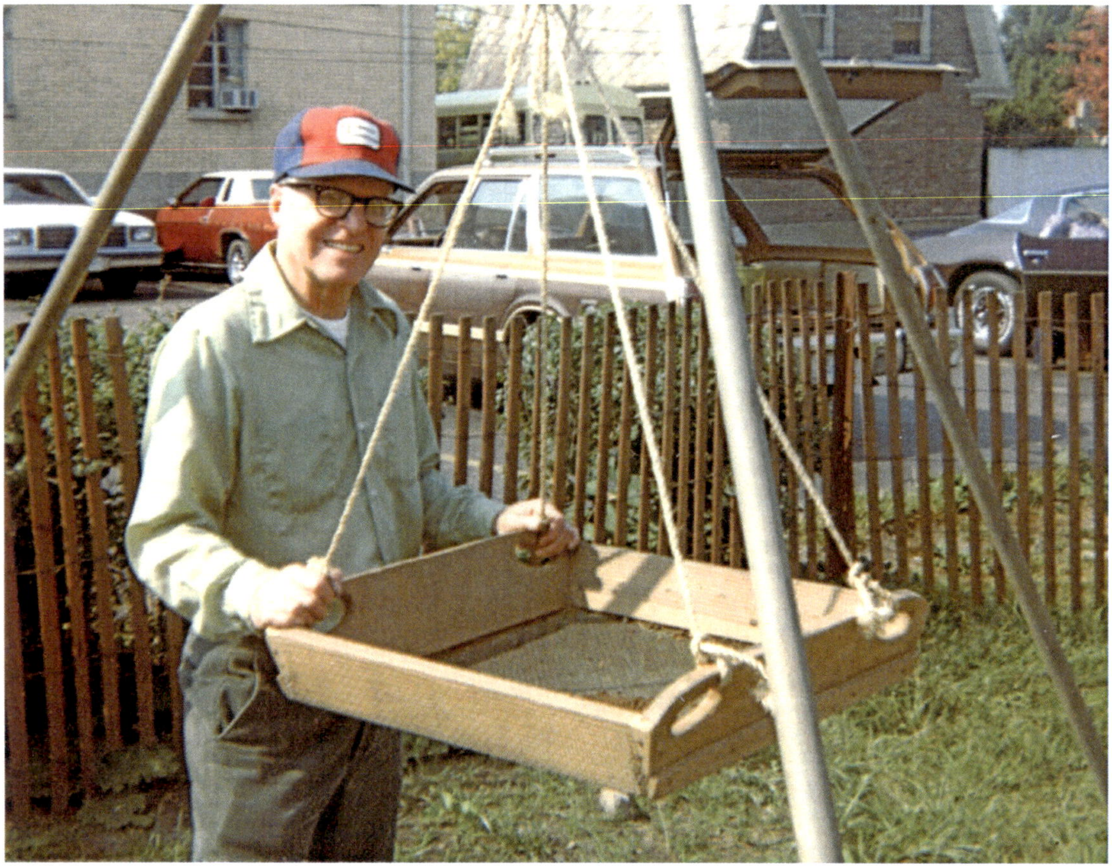

My dear friend Ernie, whose encouragement and advice, it has been my great honor and pleasure to have received, throughout a lifetime of adventures and discovery.

(Screening a Presidential home site from the early US period, 1800-1820)

1

Introduction
The Trail to the Tale

> An artifact is never the end of a story but the beginning of wonderful journey of adventure and discovery.

Artifacts by the thousands crowd shelves and display cases in many a museum and often their beauty cannot be denied. Collected, cataloged and preserved - objects to be feasted upon by our spirit and danced upon by our gaze.

Beyond their physical beauty, imagine for a moment that many have traversed their way through time with secret tales that could sweep you off your feet. What are these tales? Why are they not known? Can these artifacts lead us to associated adventures? Where are these stories?

Purchasing an artifact can be rewarding, surely the value may increase, but has the picture in the sand already been erased? Well, you say, we know who the prior owners were and that tells a tale or two. Is that so? Did these owners actually use the artifact - was one the manufacturer, salesman, tradesman, or finder of the artifact?

A list of prior owners is merely a catalog of an artifact's temporary storage over time. This is sometimes incorrectly called provenience.

Provenience is far more – most importantly it includes the "finder's statement". A "Finder" is not an archaeologist who later researches or assembles field artifacts – nor is it an archaeologist, who may have been present but did not dig up the artifacts. It is the actual "onsite" person who digs the artifacts in layer and states the associative context in their own words.

For it is at the discovery scene, like a crime scene, that the trail to the tale has the most clues. Usually stretching off in all directions, touching frontiers hardly imagined. Artifact "*associations*" form a path to the truth of things – "*surveys*" set a stage - and a "*finder's experience*" spreads a light over the scene. Validity is thus insured.

If they exist, "*original source documents*", (OSD), are the actual grains of truth, breathing life back into an artifact. Referenced documents should rarely be used. Only after verifying all supporting original source documents should referenced material be used. A certification should be included, substantially to this effect, as I do now:

> All supporting references are from original source documents - such as directories, newspapers, journals, letters, and magazines - printed or written prior to 1890. All original source documents can be identified in the bibliography by the code, OSD.
>
> Any reference to third party written material, after 1900, is not in support of the archaeological or historical context herein set forth. It is kept to an absolute minimum to avoid any appearance to the contrary.

2 Period Context - *Philadelphia - Early 1800's*
Current Context – *Philadelphia – Early 2000's*

Is it really more fulfilling to live in a more intense archeological area such as Egypt, China, Europe, India, or South America?

The fact remains that we are usually confined by our circumstances in life, despite our steady gaze over the fence suggesting the grass is so much greener in our neighbor's yard. Part of being an adult is making the best of things and finding the potential that is within our grasp.

In Eastern North America, Indian artifacts have cultural tales to tell stretching back thousands of years. Geologic fossilized artifacts are similar to those found throughout the world and have similar mysteries here as elsewhere. The fact is that the archeological history in the US has a rich history of unanswered mysteries that each of us can participate in discovering if we so wish. The key factors needed for success are determination and perseverance.

In the following pages the mysteries discussed are limited to our Eastern US region and confined by our resources to the early period of US events (*full historic interactions*) and whose effects are found by following the trail to our present time.

So here we are in Philadelphia with a trail of crumbs thick with tales of adventure. Independence National Park has been overrun with experts claiming millions of artifacts recovered and many labs working under their direction to preserve and unravel Philadelphia and national "*full historic interactions*". But Philadelphia, Boston, New York, Baltimore, Washington D.C. and so may more places, are so much more – with plenty of questions to be answered and plenty of tales missed by those who should know better.

Mental preparation is essential. We must be able to recognize important artifacts on sight, at the site, and find the initial questions each poses to start our trail to the tale. Otherwise our tale will slip from our grasp and possibly never be seen. The clues lead from crumb to crumb – rarely to direct and immediate answers. Often our peers (collectors, dealers, and archaeologists) are simply content to list, catalog, value, and view artifacts without ever seeing more than a mere one percent of the tale. Artifacts are rarely isolated in time, place, or association - this "***context***" is the soul of our artifact and provides the factual foundation on which the tale begins.

Herein, our artifact time period ("***context***") is centered in the pre civil war years stretching from colonial years through the years just before the American Civil War. Our site surveys ("***context***") are confined by our life circumstances primarily to the Philadelphia area. Our artifact associations ("***context***") are discovered during recovery and depend solely upon the skill of the finder.

Often the "finder" will benefit from constructing a classic archaeological typology. It is a statistical usage and contextual relationship map or diagram of the artifacts the finder recovered – typically various types of pottery if the site involved a period of human history. The "finder" can then examine further mysteries by integrating the local site's typology into the larger picture - spanning across many archeological sites and environments which bracket the suspected period of use.

Thus, in archaeology, experience alone does not translate to field skill. The ability to disregard pre-conceived ideas, "analysis skill", is the foundational talent needed. When this skill is present the trail to the tale will be revealed and thunder down through the ages to our current time, place, and associations ("***current context***").

An artifact's effect through time is then revealed and its message evolves, as if a circular ripple across geographic regions ("***full history***"). Looking at this complete picture we can then see if the lofty status of "*national treasure*" should be attached to our tale. Most important however is the individual fulfillment that comes from the satisfaction of navigating the maze of clues and capturing our answers – thus contributing to the great human experiment going forward.

3 Artifacts - Starting Our Journey to Discovery
(Pictures, Archeological Context, and Provenience)

In Philadelphia we are fortunate to have some detailed written records which drive our site survey. Because of this we can rapidly react to evolving situations. Rarely will anyone hand you a site – you must survey, survey, and survey again. Serious recovery activity should not be considered until this survey work is undertaken. Often pride, greed, and peer pressure result in poorly conducted recovery operations regardless of whether amateur or professional.

"*Salvage archaeology*" is a term often thrown about as an excuse to cover up poorly conducted work – often with little or no survey, screening, or associative context recorded. In my experience, all salvage operations, even after completion, offer opportunities for discovery and investigation. Again it is critically important for the finder to assemble the artifacts and their associative information. It should be recorded while memories are fresh, even if site time does not allow – do it later, but as soon as possible. Professionals often rely on students and paid companies to maintain site information and later find it is useless, looting of the site has occurred, and information manufactured to cover it up.

Often we find archaeological summaries going on and on about how similar one site is to another and therefore bypassed. Of course this is nonsense – it assumes answers before having seen the questions. How can one know what could have arisen without looking? My experience is that every site has a unique story to tell no matter how similar they may seem. You may have to work longer, harder, and differently to see each story.

Pictures, even a few, are sufficient to preserve the site context and physical layout. Often conditions are impossible (weather, light, etc.) – one should simply return when it is possible but before all is lost. In my experience rarely has all been lost when a return to a site is timely.

This is where our journey begins. A thread emerges leading to our tale. A "*national treasure*" is rarely known before some enlightened discovery. Of course exceptions are recorded – such as disasters and the resulting written inventory of losses (treasures). These treasure locations are usually ship wrecks, well known by ocean archaeologists and treasure hunters.

The thread that starts our tale is an artifact (as is it usually is). Our site, in this case was surveyed prior to a large construction project by myself for more than a year. Ultimately I obtained permission from the owner, excavation contractor and general contractor to work in an agreed manner during the project. None of this was easy and usually for the private archaeologist – impossible. My efforts were rewarded however. My site survey revealed numerous businesses and residences spanning a period from the late colonial until the present. Among the businesses were several hotels and restaurants, primarily in the years 1800 through 1900. I mapped the areas – produced weather protected site maps and noted the most probable areas for artifact recovery. I studied early directories and business ownership including other relatives of the owners (often in the same business at other locations - later answering associative questions that arise).

One must also protect the site from those who fail to obtain permission and were primarily motivated by greed. This resulted in several confrontations and some near arrests by the present owners.

The professional archaeological groups and organizations showed no interest in my site. This is not unusual because they rarely have the resources to pursue the great number of sites available.

Educated as a scientist (Physicist), I continually refined my maps and measurements as I uncovered the factual information about the site (error analysis). My models were accurate most of the time. The site was empty of buildings so no traces were evident at the surface. Slowly I worked from one end of the site through the summer, into the fall, and finally the winter before completing my work. The construction was never held up nor impacted by my work. This is critical if you plan to maintain a good working relationship with a contractor, owner, and excavator.

Rather than explain every little detail, we will focus on the details that resulted in our tale here. In early October, rain was drizzling on and off. On this day I started investigating a key area for artifacts - likely location for one of the corner hotel's privy shafts and/or wells (due to the age). It was very quiet, when around 2:30PM I uncovered the dirt over large cap stones. These in turn covered a 6 foot diameter brick lined privy shaft. The cap stones were already 7 feet under the surface covering the entire brick lined privy shaft. I removed each large blue granite stone. There were five stones, each approximately 10 feet long, 6-8 inches thick, and approximately 15-18 inches wide. After removing them with heavy equipment, I started following the trail of artifacts, layer by layer as is normal in these shafts.

In this case I was fortunate because there were no missing layers due to periodic cleaning or final closing of the privy. The age started in the late 1880's, progressing next to 1870's next 1860's, next 1850's, next 1840's, next 1830's, and next 1820's and finally 1810 - 1800 (25 feet deep).

The lower layers were primarily heavy black silt often found in deep, North American, city privies. The bottom 5 feet consisted of this heavy black privy silt in which many artifacts are embedded. It blocks all oxygen and traps everything like glue. However over the years one can develop careful techniques to peal it away and expose the artifacts. If you decide to screen the black silt layer, it must be water screened because of its glue like consistency.

Embedded in the black silt, at approximately 23 feet, is where our artifact was found – in a layer well under the typical blue Staffordshire pottery of the mid 1820's and well under the freehand flower drawn "folkware" pottery of the early 1820's. All preliminary indications at the time of recovery (on site) - from its associative context - suggest a period of use around 1815 to 1820.

Our artifact is an oval (egg) shaped light green bottle. It has raised lettering horizontally across the body of the bottle stating "Cullen's / Patent / Liquid / Magnesia". It is immediately wrapped in the hole and removed to special safety storage on my vehicle on site. Both temperature and humidity are duplicated and it is gradually brought to surface conditions over the next few days. These storage devices are extremely simple to make (on site) during the actual recovery process. One professional dig I know of - the archeologists placed their recovered artifacts neatly lined up on the surface ground without protection and then later drove their vehicle over them – crushing all. Enough said.

The work on site continues until midnight – mostly in the cold rain (around 40 degrees). The importance of having protective gear cannot be stressed enough because once your hands or feet are wet – the dig for you will be over quickly. Hard hats are essential. Massive gear and tools are unnecessary – keep it simple and small as possible then your attention can be focused on recovery. As in deep ocean archaeology – unless you have nerves of steel – always have a partner who is awake and focused no matter what the conditions. In my 35 years of experience I only know of two archaeologists, capable of working alone in deep water (150 feet or deeper), or in deep land shafts (15 to 40 feet). Do not try it – you will get hurt.

If time and resources are unlimited, try to dig in fair weather. Professional sites are typically massive undertakings with a well defined bureaucracy. Often the least experienced are the finders (students or minimum wage laborers) – the leading professionals are often not seen except to claim publication rights and attend media events. In the United States there are no partnerships between the amateurs, professionals, collectors, and antique dealers. This is regrettable because we are losing our artifact context and tales, on a massive scale. In Europe and most of the rest of the world exactly the opposite is true. England has, for more than 150 years, a partnership between these groups - with great respect and sharing among them. As a respected US Archaeologist from Philadelphia said to me on many occasions, such a partnership was his most important wish going forward. I can recall his counsel, respect for my independence, and visits to many of my sites with great fondness – he is indeed missed. (*See commented and emphasized quote below*)

John Cotter, an eminent archaeologist from Philadelphia and professor at "*University of Pennsylvania*" for almost four decades - dedicated his life to establishing American historical and cultural archaeology at a professional level. This included reaching out to his colleagues to accept a partnership with independent archaeologists and other interested layman and groups, as John's quoted statement below from four decades earlier discloses.

"… Solutions that will save a maximum of historic sites are simple in theory, expensive in practice, and often impractical in fact. Even when limited funds are finally gathered for archaeological salvage, there looms a dearth of trained archaeologists. Many willing groups of amateurs exist who may take pleasure and pride in contributing their services gratis or for essential expenses, but they must be competently led, and the professional is called upon to contribute his services when he is often paid no more that the junior grades of landscape architects, planners, and engineers whose services are devoted to altering the landscape. Yet the intelligent cooperation of the amateur archaeologist remains the best hope of nourishing the cause of conservation and reminding elected office-holders of the national duty to preserve the story of the past. The informed and interested layman and the professional archaeologist here join hands in a common effort….." *(By John Cotter)*

His statement clearly supports my position which I stated earlier at the beginning of this work and I repeat here again:

Archaeology is for everyone, everywhere, and surrounds all of us in our daily lives. Competent independent archaeologists and amateurs will continue to flourish making significant contributions of first impression.

The work of independents will be used and cited by professionals who will continue to decline any meaningful partnership. However John maintained personal links to those of us in the independent arena over these many decades, hoping for our acceptance by his peers and institutions. I will only comment to say, sadly, his proposals remain open after more than four decades and his passing on February 5, 1999.

So, now we have our artifact pictures - the context is preserved and the provenience started. The adventure begins. Illumination will start with a thread – a crumb – as we begin weaving our way to the truth of things. Our tale will come alive.

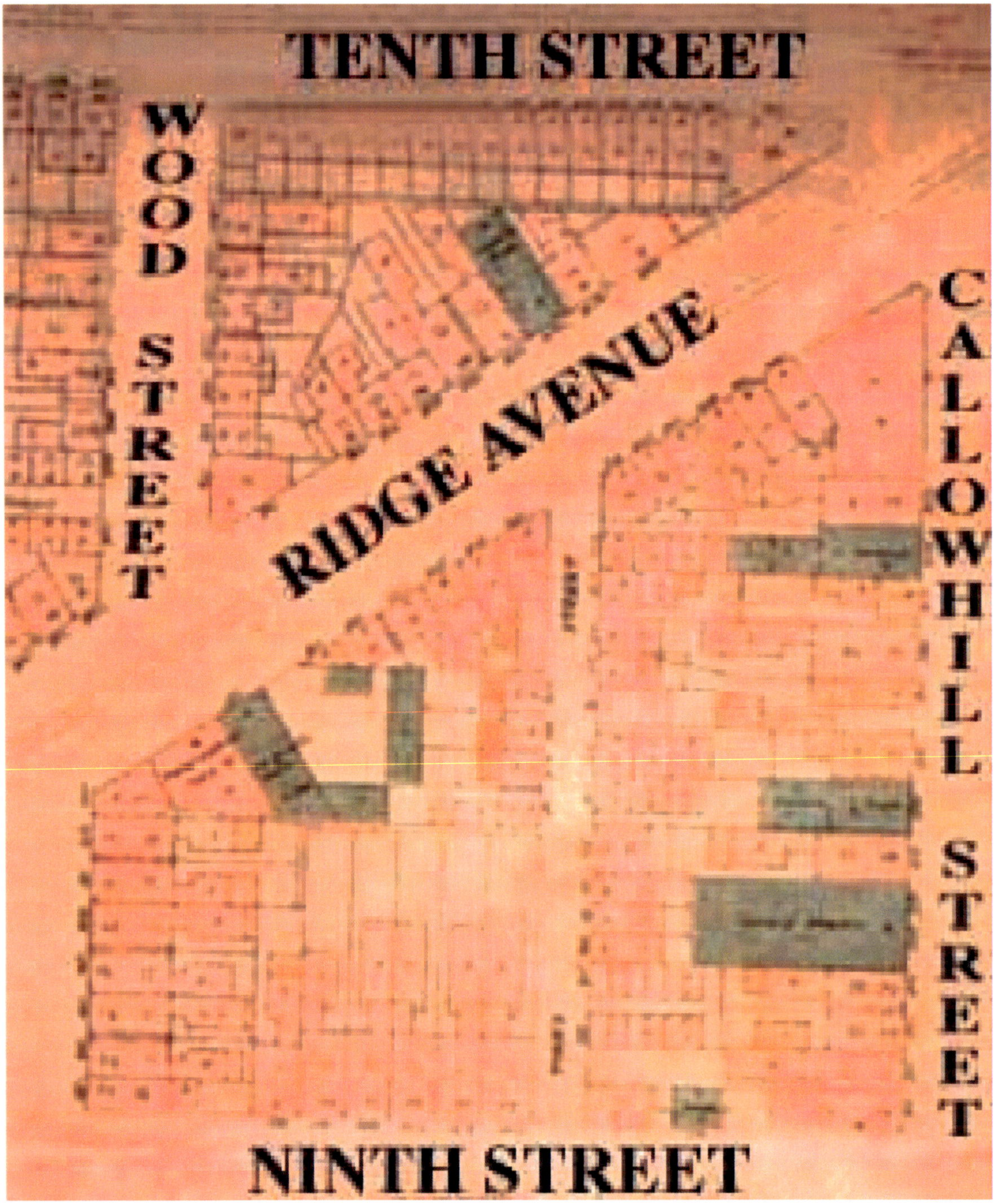

One of many site maps I used from May 2004 through December 2005. My work on site was in coordination with the construction manager so I followed their schedule - a process of go slow then fast. Rarely is the timing ideal. My actual digging started in May 2005. I completed site work by December 2005. This map is an original source document, (OSD) and dates from approximately 1858 – 1859. (*Commonly known to both professionals and amateurs - Hexamer & Locher pre-Civil War Philadelphia Map series – Courtesy Free Library of Philadelphia)*

(Continued on next page)

Site surveying is essential. In Philadelphia we are fortunate to have a wealth of written historic materials. After your site inspection and any rough drawings are made – weather proof your site maps. You will need it for reference more than you can imagine. Things do not always go according to plan and you will need your error analysis skills mentioned earlier. I've known many people, professional and amateur over the years, who have missed important sites they should have discovered. I have always owed a debt of thanks to them for their unselfish and unknown kindness to me.

This particular map shows more than 50 years of building and street changes from before the Civil War. Combined with knowledge of the street changes as shown in Appendix E - the oldest part of the construction site should be the buildings facing Ridge Ave. This fact was confirmed by archaeological evidence dug over the entire site and the presence of hidden water wells on the Ridge Avenue properties. No water wells were found on properties facing Wood Street, where it cuts (going west) through Ridge Avenue.

The water wells appeared to have been closed around 1815 – 1820 and then used as a trash repository for four decades. This corresponds to when Wood Street was expanded across Ridge Avenue around 1817 – 1818. (Appendix E)

The construction techniques used when building the "*water wells and privy shafts*" for Ridge Avenue properties, were consistent with those used in the late 18th and very early 19th century (before running water). The wells and privies were often constructed within five to ten feet of each other. Of course this meant the privy water moved to the well before being cleansed by percolation layers and many became sick after drinking the water. This construction technique was further justified because the open ground remaining on most lots was small and the adjoining back property areas bunched together as they are here on this site. Thus, bottled mineral water and spirits were popular in taverns and hotels to avoid getting sick (as well as to recover if you got sick). Of course poorly preserved food was a common problem which required mineral water to settle one's stomach as well.

Although the "*Philadelphia City Water Works*" was started in 1801/1802, in took some time before water pipes were installed in the streets throughout the city. After the transition to city water, well water was mostly used for outdoor cleaning or bathing purposes, rather than drinking or cooking. In modern day we have similar problems in undeveloped regions of the world.

One of the problem areas in early city water systems were the street hydrants. The solution to this problem (leaky water hydrants), has a surprising connection to the emergence of the US artificial mineral water industry and ultimately reached back to Europe as well. *(See Appendix B – Early Patents Issued in the name of James Ewing)*

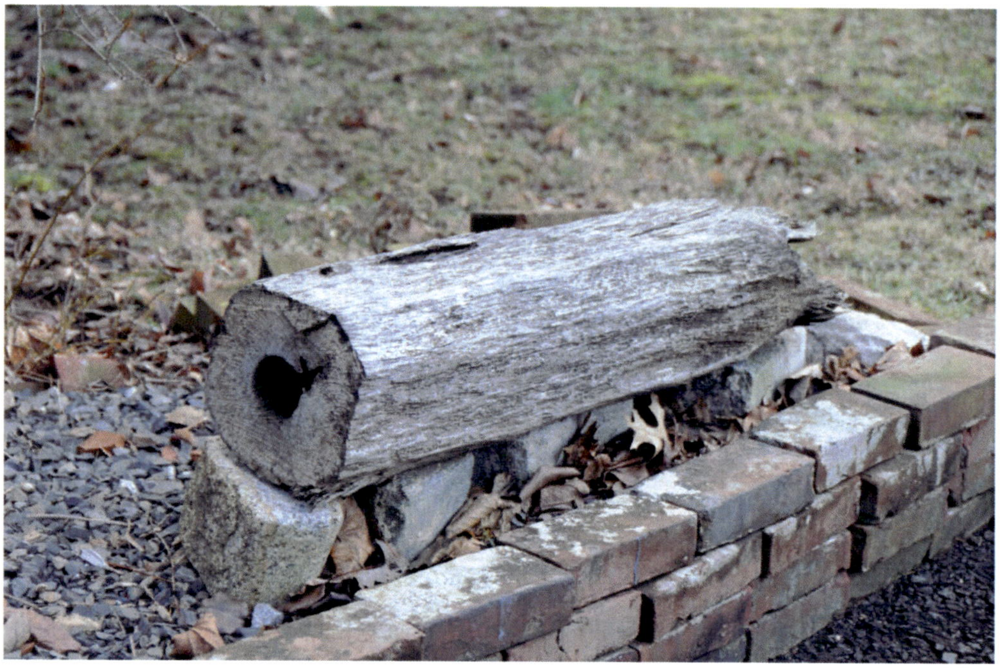

A cut cross section of a Philadelphia street water pipe from approximately 1799-1822. This small section was cut from a 25 ft. long wood pipe - similar in length to today's telephone poles. They were buried under the streets and connected end to end. The original male end can be seen at the far end. It was fitted into the female end of another wooden pole. Often the access points for individual houses were located at these joints. In 1822 wood pipes were replaced by cast iron pipes (Fairmount Waterworks -Frederick Graff).

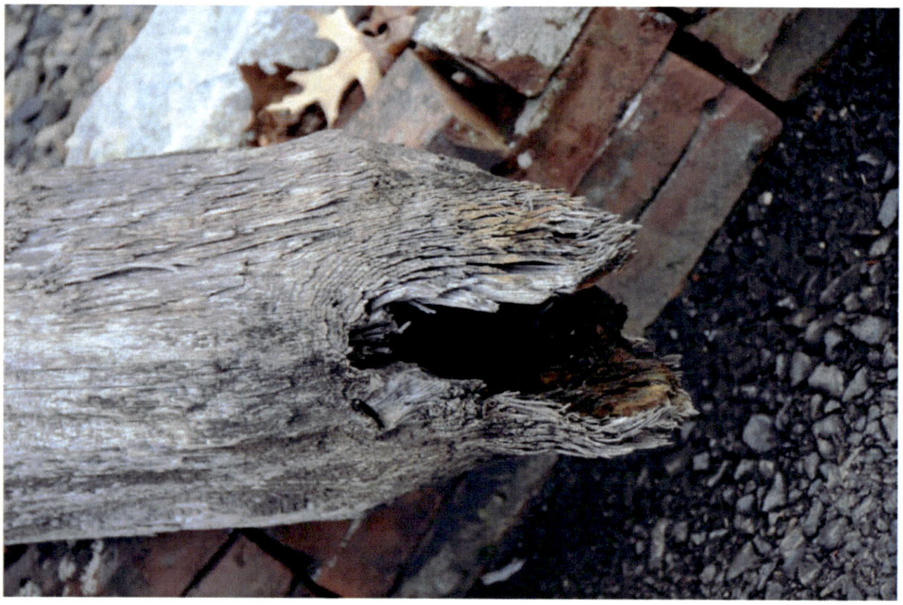

This pipe not only was taper fitted into the next pipe but also contained an early style access point. The iron residue can be seen from this local service that was inserted perpendicularly into the slot above. The slotted joint not only allowed for local access but it formed a pressure fitted joint to the next pipe in the street. You will notice there is no iron residue in the central pipe channel except at the access point. Also, the iron residue is deposited in only one direction.

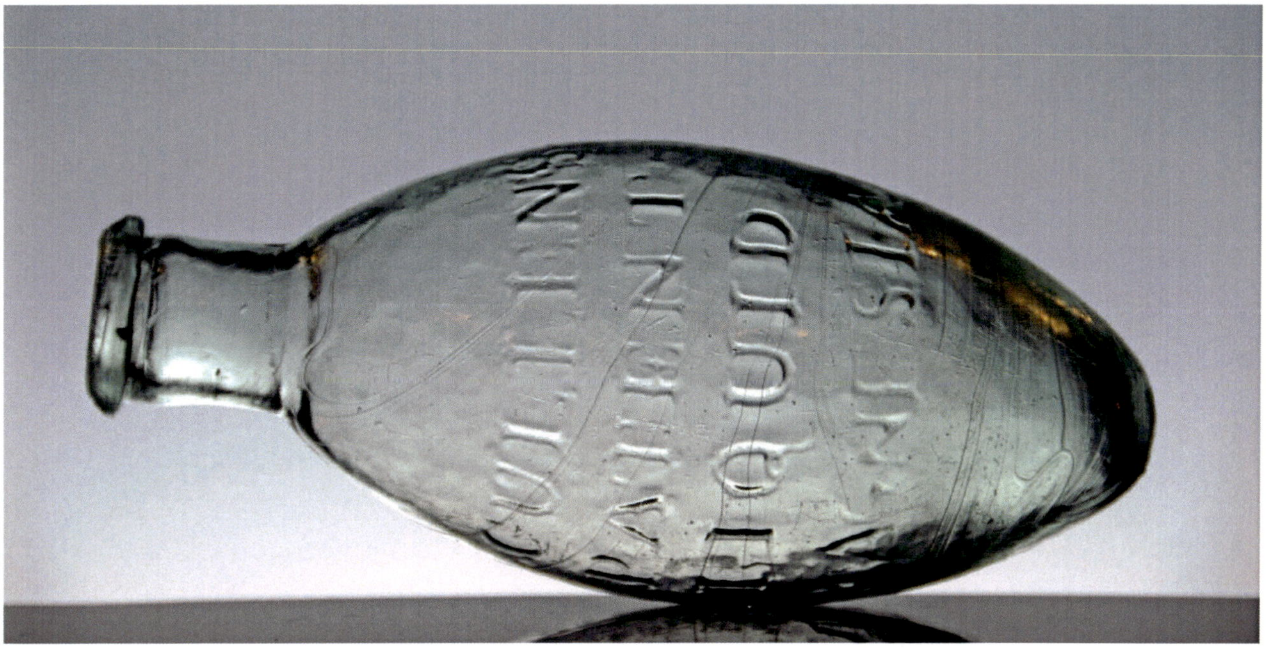

"Cullen's Patent Liquid Magnesia" April 1818 – December 1818
Hand formed, sheared neck, ¼' string glass ring around neck.
Approximately ½ pint capacity - Artifact is pictured near its natural color
(Size - 6 1/8 in high by 2 11/16 in diameter at the center)
US LETTERS PATENT Granted MAY 4, 1818

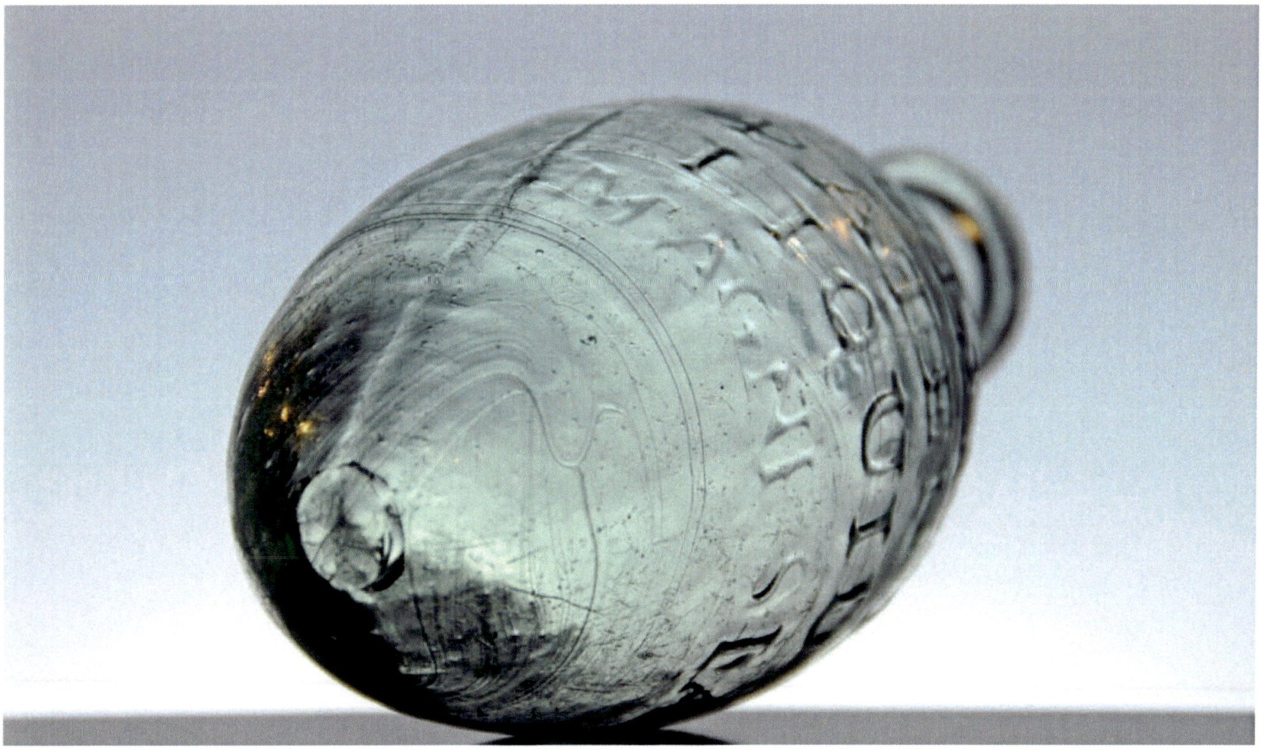

Round bottom with open ring pontil - Pictured as recovered

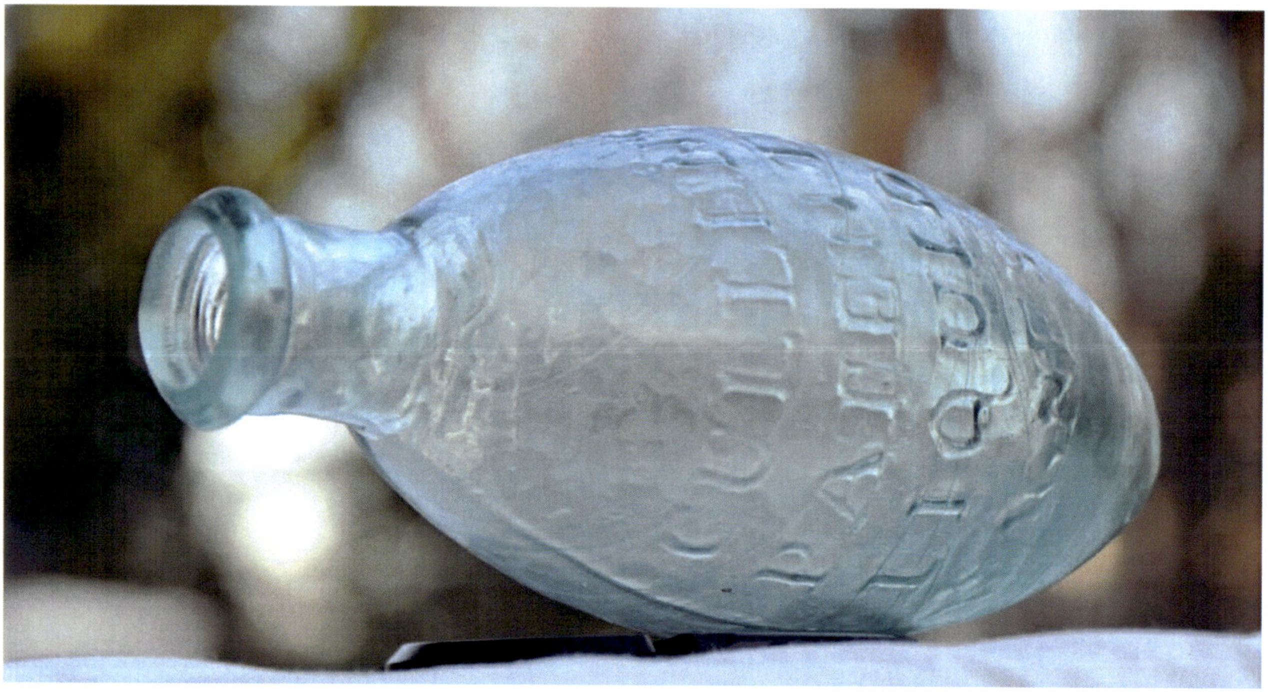

Color is distorted in these photographs - Actual color is light green.

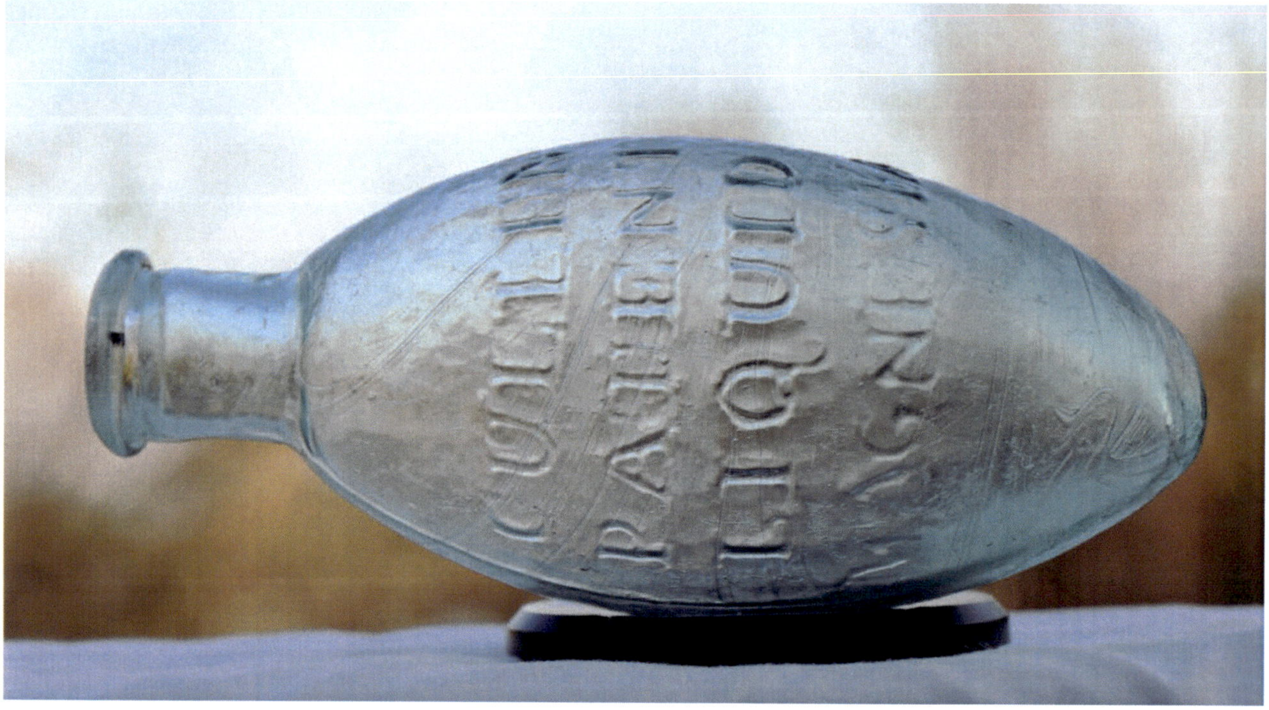

Artifact is pictured as recovered except for color – Not restored, cleaned, or altered.

City Ordinances—List of Penalties.

For wasting the Schuylkill water 5 dollars
Empty boxes remaining in the street longer than 3 hours 1 dollar 33 cents
Goods remaining in do. more than 4 hours 2 dollars
Occupying stands in the market unappropriated by ordinance 2 dollars
Exposiag goods for sale on or over the brick or stone pavement 1 dollar 33 cents
For persons remaining in the market after market hours 5 dolls
Riding or driving immoderately 3 dollars
Driving without reins and without being within reach of the horse's head 3 dollars
Riding or driving on or over the brick or stone pavement, except going into a stable or enclosure 5 dollars
Piling lumber or unloding out of a cart, &c. any bar iron, coal, &c. on the footway 5 dollars
Hackney coaches not numbered as the law directs 5 dollars.
Drays and carts do. 10 dollars

Acts of Assembly.

Selling ardent or vinous spirits within the city or county of Philadelphia, by less measure than one quart, without having a license 50 dollars for the first offence, and 100 dollars for every subsequent transgression. By a late act of assembly, any respectable citizen is made a competent witness. The fine is to be applied to the use of the poor.
Chimnies being on fire, not having been swept within one calender month 5 dollars 33 cents
Throwing privy filth in the street 4 dollars,

Whitley's Philadelphia Register for 1820 - Part of Page XCIII
City Ordinances and Penalties

Above is a list of Philadelphia's laws and fines for causing public nuisances, such as throwing privy filth in the street, $4, or wasting the Schuylkill water, $5. These were the local laws in effect when John Cullen lived and worked in Philadelphia – also possibly when his mineral water was used at the "*tavern – hotel*" near the corner of Ridge Road & Wood Street in 1818. Public water was clearly available by 1820 as the law above suggests. Losing control of your horse was not a good idea, $3 - nor was shorting a customer on the volume of a bottle of porter or liquor, $50 for first offense.

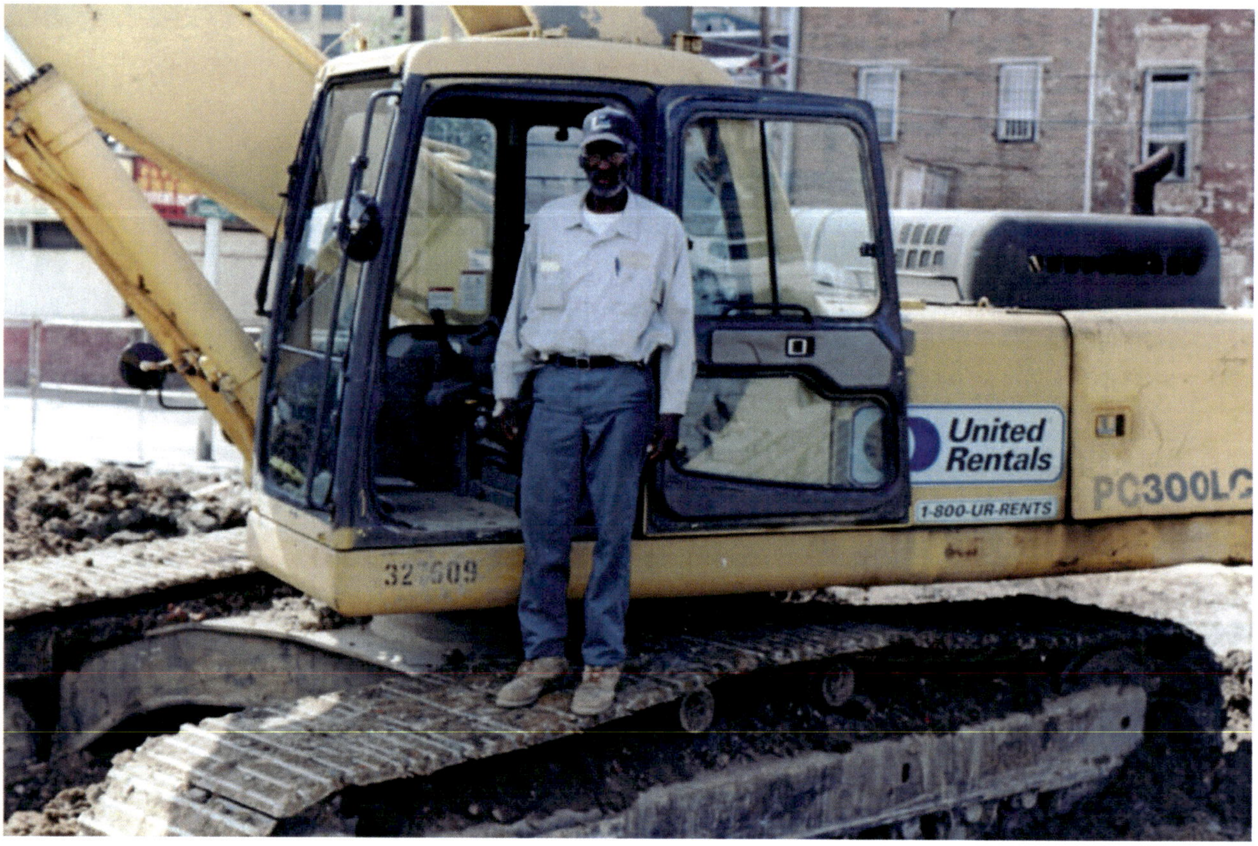

Heavy equipment is often necessary, as I mentioned in the previous chapter. Here my dear friend Sam poses with equipment that is used when necessary. Many sites of significant importance to our national historic past in Philadelphia would have been destroyed and lost forever without wonderful people such as Sam.

The City of Philadelphia owns an enormous debt of gratitude to these people, who give of their time, money, and heart, to the city's future thru its past. Sam is an example of a terrific role model who we can all learn from. The quiet strength of Sam, his Company, and his family are what makes American great.

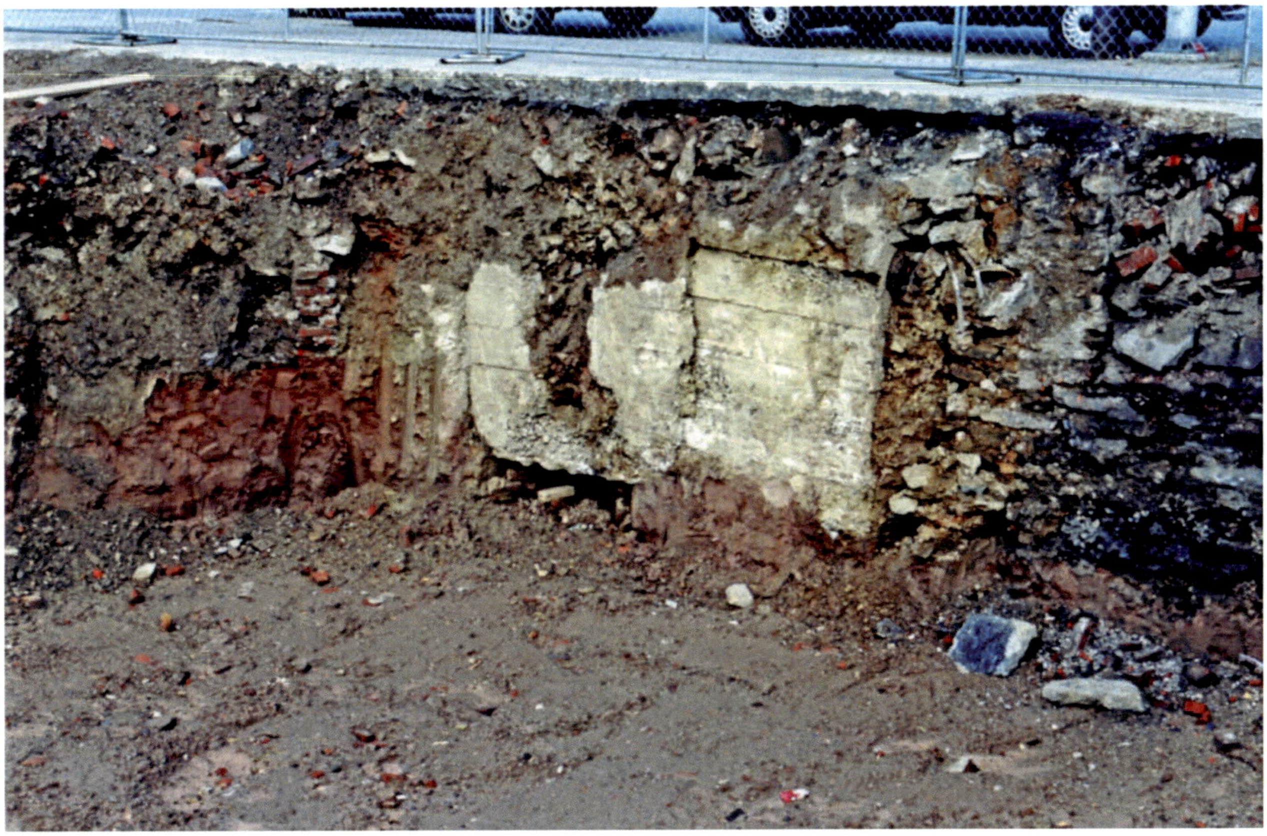

Recovery site showing the actual level where large cap stones were found and removed by heavy equipment pictured on the previous page. The large concrete block in the center of the picture marks the end of a privy line. All were removed as part of the construction project and would have been lost without the permission of owners, site managers, excavators, general contractors, and inspectors.

All privies were brick lined and varied in diameter and depth. In this privy line, three privies were 6 feet in diameter, two were 5 ½ feet in diameter, one was 4 feet in diameter. Three privy lines were found on this site – each with similar number of privy shafts, although most were only 15 feet deep.

The end privy of the pictured privy line is shown under the concrete block in the center of the picture. It was 4 feet in diameter and was initially a well and later used as a privy when city water became available – it was 25 feet deep. Three were 25 feet deep, two 20 feet, and one 15 feet. Only one had capstones. The earliest building foundations varied in age from approximately 1800 – 1820. One large cold cellar existed with brick drainage channels under a brick floor. The cold cellar had street entry for delivery of barrels and boxes of perishables, typically used in restaurants and hotels of that period. An embossed wooden beer barrel tap was recovered which correlated to the historical records of the 1840 -1860 period. Ice handling tools were recovered as well.

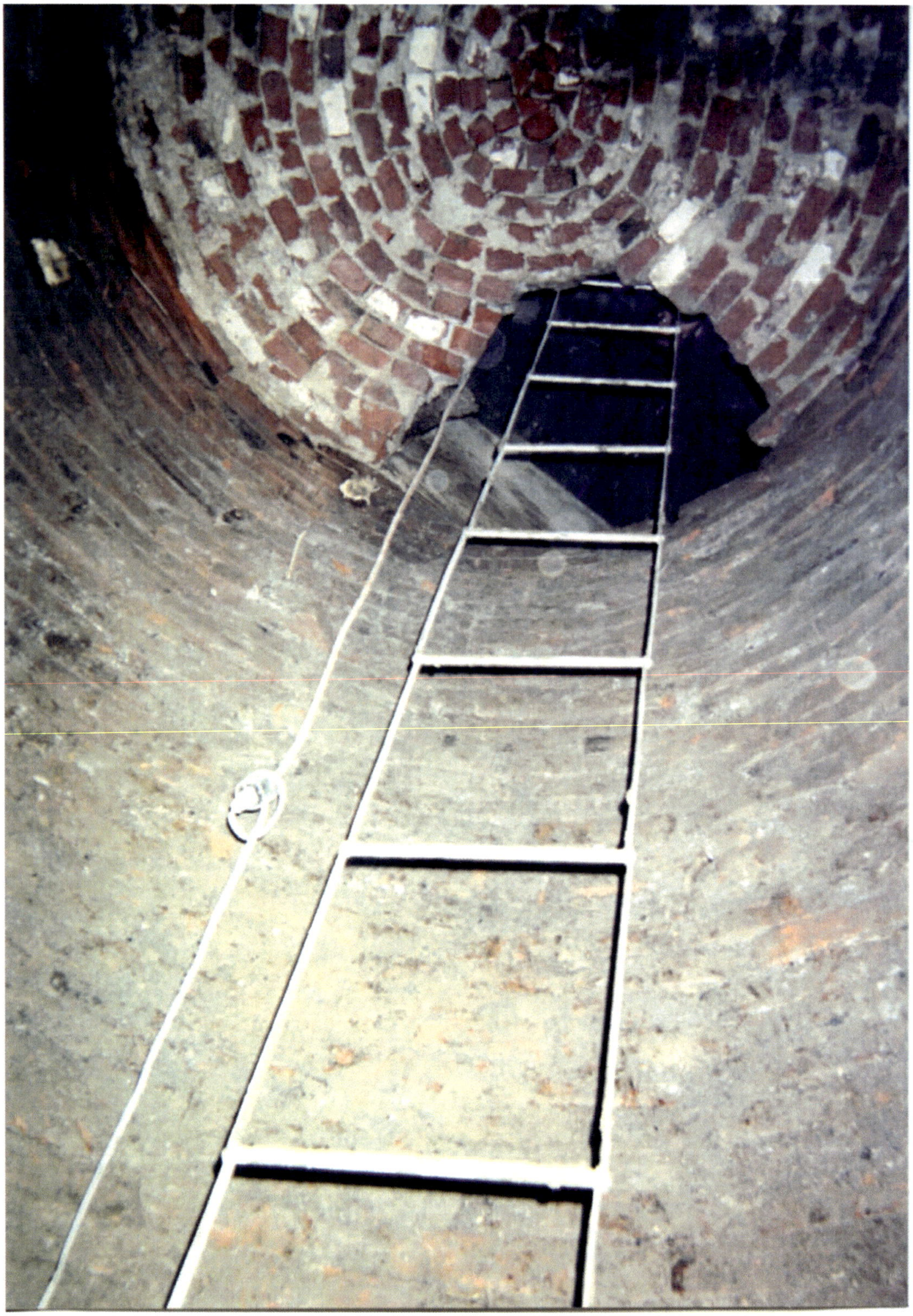

This picture is taken looking up from approximately the 10 foot level of a 25 foot deep Philadelphia privy shaft. The diameter is 5 ½ feet, slightly smaller than the actual recovery shaft which was 6 feet. Also the cap here is a 20th century cemented brick dome, whereas in the recovery shaft it was long flat blue granite cap stones, side by side over the entire top.

4 Building from Absolute Facts to Theory (Similar to CSI)

What are the **facts** (crumbs/threads) that will lead us to illumination?

- ***Shape, size, and color – the physical appearance of the artifact.***
- ***Context age of the artifact by associative artifacts.***
- ***The raised words and lettering on the artifact.***
- ***Found in a Hotel privy used in the early period of US history.***
- ***Location of the site (city, state, region, street, etc.).***
- ***Associated artifacts – (yardsticks - i.e. pottery).***
- ***Manufacturing marks – (open pontil, crude sheared lip with applied glass string below it).***
- ***The bottle was made in a custom mold, for Cullen exclusively.***
- ***Other artifacts bearing the name Cullen from the mid 19th century.***

Not much to start with except that its shape is unusual – especially if it's associative context (age) is confirmed somehow.

What initial question(s) do these facts (crumbs) raise to start us on our journey of discovery? Of course, some are easier to answer than others.

- ***Is the artifact domestic or foreign in origin?***
- ***Where was the artifact made?***
- ***Who made the artifact? (What company?)***
- ***Does the raised lettering lead us to any historical records?***
- ***Are the associated artifacts, dug with this bottle, of a known age?***
- ***Are the associated artifacts consistent in age with this one?***
- ***Are there other artifacts with the name "Cullen" related to our artifact?***
- ***Are the artifact's characteristics (color, weight, lip style, etc.) similar to artifacts of known local origin? If so what glasshouses?***
- ***Is the artifact a product of the Hotel's owners or managers?***

We can answer the last question with some certainty due to my preliminary site survey information (taken from historical documents covering the site's timeline of use). Clearly, the artifact's raised lettering does not match the name of any known hotel owner or manager in the timeline of use.

One must always adjust, should later evidence suggest a different answer to a question. Good error analysis will uncover the truth. So don't worry at this stage if you are later corrected by your research.

Often it is desirable to consult a trusted friend who is also an expert or peer, and pose a question. Although you may have an idea as to the answer – other's opinions should be solicited as a self-checking mechanism. In this case I posed the question as to "domestic or foreign in origin?" to such a friend. I suspected strongly from my own experience the artifact was domestic but the word "PATENT" was uncommon on domestic artifacts of this type and suspected age. My friend confirmed my theory that the egg bottle appears to be domestic in origin. Of course, more evidence will be needed to either confirm or deny this preliminary theory.

All the associated artifacts in layer with the artifact under investigation were of the time period 1800 through 1820. Early pottery shards were the primary associated artifacts although some glass and carved bone were found as well.

In archaeology, pottery shards are the yardstick commonly used to identify a period of time in human history. Most regions, cultures, and time periods have their own unique pottery. In prehistoric periods, trilobite fossils are used to identify the age of associated fossils which are not as well known or unique. Like pottery, trilobites are unique within time periods. These are two of the common yardsticks used – others exist as well. Of course scientific testing for selected atomic level isotopes can further refine and confirm your artifact's age determination (such as carbon 14 testing used with organic based artifacts, etc.)

The remaining questions arise from the artifact itself - The raised lettering "Cullen's / Patent / Liquid / Magnesia" and the appearance (color, shape etc.).

The raised lettering indicates the bottle was blown in a custom mold – for Cullen exclusively. The bottle shows no evidence of a mold slug plate or ghosted lettering (hammered out for reuse by Cullen). Therefore the mold was likely made expressly for Cullen in response to an order from him. Who that manufacturer is, remains an open question to be answered later.

The word "***Patent***" on domestic artifacts of this age and type is somewhat unusual, maybe unique. Perhaps it is a foreign patent on a domestic bottle such as exists on "*Turlington*" or "*Essence*" bottles of the early US period. Regardless, I will need to verify if it is an actual US patent or not. So the trail leads me to United States patent records. Unfortunately, prior to 1836 all patent records were destroyed in a fire. However various patent indexes were not. Some basic minimal information remains identifying approximately 10,000 patents of which approximately 2800 have been reconstructed since 1836. These patents are known as the X patents because they were not numbered until after the great fire of 1836. Information about such a patent is likely unknown. After hunting around for some time I locate a searchable list (not all, but between 1790 and 1829). *(See "Patent" analysis information in Appendixes A & B.)*

My search leads me through wonderful history and I begin to feel it speaking to me through these records. They are little understood even by the experts and patent office officials. The records are listed by date in ascending order, after sorting by last name I discover one "Cullen". Next I notice the description (title of the patent) which jumps out at me *"Medicated Liquid Magnesia"*. This is starting to look good. Next let's see where the patent letter was issued (sent) – what city? The index says "Philadelphia" under the name "John Cullen". This is really getting exciting! *The wording is almost exactly the same as the artifact's raised lettering! The patent issue date is May 4, 1818.* A spectacularly early date! More facts (crumbs) raising more questions as the tale is expanding.

- ***With a date and name, can we find correlation with Philadelphia directory entries? Do any even exist?***
- ***Are there other possible historical records in Philadelphia from this time period? Newspapers, magazines, letters, journals, etc?***

Searching year by year forward from 1799 through 1860 we find "John Cullen" listed in a very narrow range of years. His occupation is consistent with the artifact but then his address and occupation suddenly change after two years. After another three years he disappears completely.

Year	Listed Name	Philadelphia Address	Occupation	Ref
1811	(not listed)			49
1813	(not listed)			46
1814	(not listed)			50
1816	(not listed)			49
1817	(not listed)			49
1817	(not listed)			47
1818	Cullen, John	NE cor. Chestnut and 2nd Sts.	Chymist & c.	46
1819	Cullen, John	NE cor. Chestnut and 2nd Sts.	Chemist & c.	46
1820	Cullen, John	92 S Front St.	MD, Chemist & c.	36
1821	Cullen, John	92 S Front St.	MD, Chemist & c.	51
1822	Cullen, John	92 S Front St.	MD, Chemist & c.	51
1823	(not listed)			2
1824	(not listed)			2
1825	(not listed)			37
1828	(not listed)			2
1829	(not listed)			2
1830	(not listed)			2
1831	(not listed)			2
1833	(not listed)			2
1835	(not listed)			2
1837	(not listed)			2
1839	(not listed)			1
1840	(not listed)			1
1841	(not listed)			1
1842	(not listed)			1

1843	(not listed)			1
1844	(not listed)			1

A whole series of new questions arise from these facts (crumbs).

- ***Where did John Cullen come from before living in Philadelphia?***
- ***Where did John Cullen disappear to?***
- ***Did he pass away?***
- ***Did he suddenly discontinue his drug business to become a MD?***
- ***Did he get a Medical Degree from a Philadelphia school?***
- ***Did he just add the "MD" title to his name?***
- ***Did anyone else take over his druggist chemical business?***
- ***Was his Patented "Liquid Magnesia" the only mineral water he made?***
- ***Did he advertise his patented mineral water?***
- ***Was the mineral water sold in a soda fountain as well as bottles?***
- ***Did he have other sizes of bottles?***
- ***How much did he charge for the mineral water?***
- ***Where did he obtain the bottles?***
- ***Who made the bottles?***

Additionally, we have not yet answered all the questions mentioned before these new queries arose. They must be addressed as well.

The tale now eclipses the beauty of the artifact and the story of its recovery. The artifact is acquiring its own voice – speaking to us – enriching our lives and establishing a historical framework going forward. The trail is laid before us. The threads wend their way through time forward and backward.

So let's continue.

5 John Cullen and his Historical Context

We now have our character established and a beginning of our historical context with patent office index records and Philadelphia directory entries. One of the threads leading from the directory entries is John Cullen's occupation of MD in 1820 through 1822. It's not likely we will find anything because pharmacists in the early period of US history could easily add MD to their name. License requirements did not come about until many years later. Also, many doctors were immigrants and if college educated, likely obtained degrees or credentials overseas.

Where will I start this process? He appears to be new to Philadelphia so it is not likely he has had time to establish any medical school relationships. The fact is, he was devoting himself to his druggist business, if directory entries in 1818 and 1819 are accurate. Even in today's world juggling such a life is difficult. But sometimes in history, a character is so strong in pursuit of his desire; he jumps out of the mists of time, bold and heroic. What appears improbable to us, as mere mortals, becomes the most probable. *Could our character be such a person?* He was savvy enough to get a patent at a very early time, when the majority of people had a limited education. *Could this be the tip of an iceberg?*

What medical schools existed in Philadelphia in 1818 – 1820? Philadelphia directories and "*As it Is – Stranger's Guides*" often included colleges and universities, as well as public schools. These list the "*University of Pennsylvania*" medical college as well as its faculty. Even at that time it was well known and the largest medical college in Philadelphia. So let's start there since it is familiar to me. Maybe we'll get lucky.

My trip to the university library system is on a beautiful early summer day. The flowers are everywhere. This alone was worth the time and energy. Libraries are generally full of wonderful, helpful people who know the structure of their systems, not necessarily details of what's in them. So it is up to you to recognize likely repositories of historical information. Often, your questions lead nowhere.

A quality I mentioned earlier that you must possess is determination. This is where that quality will be tested to its limits. The library system does not appear on first contact to have references to our character. Most large colleges such as this one have more than one main library – they often have many smaller specialized libraries. Is there a medical school library? Yes! Did I have any better luck? No! Finally, I ask myself the right question!

Is it possible early records exist in some form of archival department, not normally thought of as a library? The reference librarian answers, "Yes"! Since we are living in the 21st century I decide to try one of our cultural innovations, the internet, in order to access the archival department. We're in luck - a partial catalog exists of archived records. A search pops up an entry for a document written by John Cullen. Wow – is this our character? The entry says it's a letter to the Dean of the Medical faculty, "John Redman Coxe" requesting special allowance to obtain a "Medical Degree" based on prior experience. The entry contains a notation that John Cullen's written request was approved by a majority of the faculty. Most importantly the date of the letter is stated to be December 28, 1818. This is spectacular! The least probable story now appears to have become a fact.

Quickly, phone listings are checked and a telephone number for an archival department is found, "The University Archives and Records Center". As expected the curators are wonderful and helpful. Success does not mean you lose your head however. Now, questions will arise fast - just as it does in the middle of a scientific experiment when it is necessary to flesh out your partial differential equations to get at the truth of things (error analysis).

Since we appear to have found a fertile repository, perhaps there may be other records that will lead to more clues (crumbs) in our trail to the tale?

- ***If John Cullen was a medical student are there records – perhaps student records or alumni records?***

I ask the curators and receive a positive response – Wow! This is terrific news. Would it be possible to get copies of those records as well as the hand written letter? Yes! (This is a good day!)

The copies arrive after several anxious days and I have my first real contact with our person, "*John Cullen*". The handwritten letter is first to go under my microscope. The flow, vocabulary, and grammar give us feeling – we begin to see the man – flesh and bones - as we enter his life in December 1818. We start to discover his character. The letter is more than we could have hoped for. Direct evidence confirming his life at that time – no second hand summaries – no hearsay – no speculation – just hard undeniable facts. Fabulous!

A nice surprise is the direct confirmation of his whereabouts for a key missing year, 1817. In the letter near the end, John Cullen states:

"…..In addition to what I have stated, I trust when it be known that I have enjoyed every advantage which a resident of Eighteen Months in the Alms House of this city could afford, that the faculty will consider these various sources of obtaining information as Equivalent to a course of lectures. Respectfully awaiting this determination I have the honor to be your very obedient servant. John Cullen". ***(See pages 32 and 33 for images of John Cullen's full letter.)***

In our timeline that would place John Cullen in Philadelphia no later than June 1817. So he was running a druggist business and working at the "Alms House" too. Very busy person, but is there more? Is he also taking courses at medical school too? According to a handwritten entry in his alumni record, the date he started medical school is listed as 1816 (without a month). The date of graduation is listed as April 15, 1819. So our character between 1816 and 1819 is involved in:

- ***Working in the Philadelphia Alms house,***
- ***inventing patented products to sell,***
- ***attending a famous medical school,***
- ***and proprietor of a druggist and chemical store***

The significance of these two new documents, plus patent and directory records, is that John Cullen can be placed in Philadelphia in the years 1816 through 1821. His activity is documented by direct historical evidence. But can we determine where he came from, where he went to, and why? These questions are still remaining from earlier. We need more crumbs (clues in our trail to the tale).

We find them by analysis of the alumni records document:

- ***He was born in Dublin Ireland sometime around the year 1797,***
- ***Where he attended Trinity College,***
- ***He passed away in Richmond, Virginia December 25, 1849***
- ***He was one of the founders of the Medical College of Virginia in 1838.***

These new clues and threads are spreading in all directions - across continents and regions. This is becoming a terrific tale - with accomplishments and great deeds. We are beginning to weave the disparate parts of John Cullen's life together and the total picture is emerging. The thought occurs to me – this story is likely to continue being compiled and/or corrected for many years by other academic researchers – I am only the first of many to come. So my work here is simply a beginning.

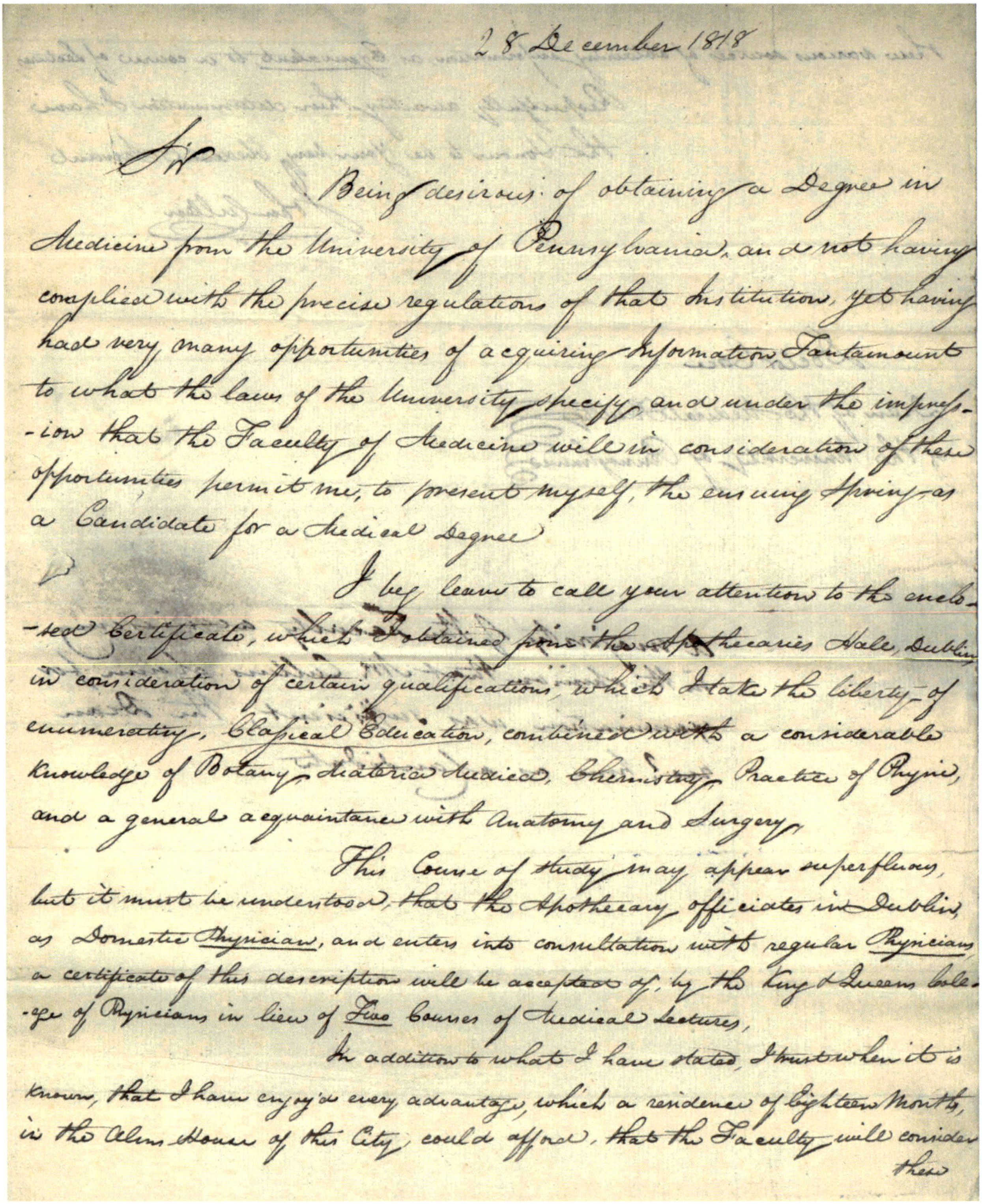

28 December 1818

Sir

Being desirous of obtaining a Degree in Medicine from the University of Pennsylvania, and not having complied with the precise regulations of that Institution, yet having had very many opportunities of acquiring Information Tantamount to what the laws of the University specify, and under the impression that the Faculty of Medicine will in consideration of these opportunities permit me, to present myself, the ensuing Spring as a Candidate for a Medical Degree

I beg leave to call your attention to the enclosed Certificate, which I obtained from the Apothecaries Hall, Dublin in consideration of certain qualifications, which I take the liberty of enumerating, Classical Education, combined with a considerable knowledge of Botany, Materia Medica, Chemistry, Practice of Physic, and a general acquaintance with Anatomy and Surgery.

This Course of study may appear superfluous, but it must be understood, that the Apothecary officiates in Dublin, as Domestic Physician, and enters into consultation with regular Physicians a certificate of this description will be accepted of, by the King & Queens College of Physicians in lieu of Two Courses of Medical Lectures,

In addition to what I have stated, I trust when it is known, that I have enjoy'd every advantage, which a residence of Eighteen Months, in the Alms House of this City, could afford, that the Faculty will consider them

Page 1: John Cullen's handwritten letter December 28, 1818
Request for Accelerated Medical Degree from U of P & Alms House statement
(From the Collections of the University of Pennsylvania Archives)

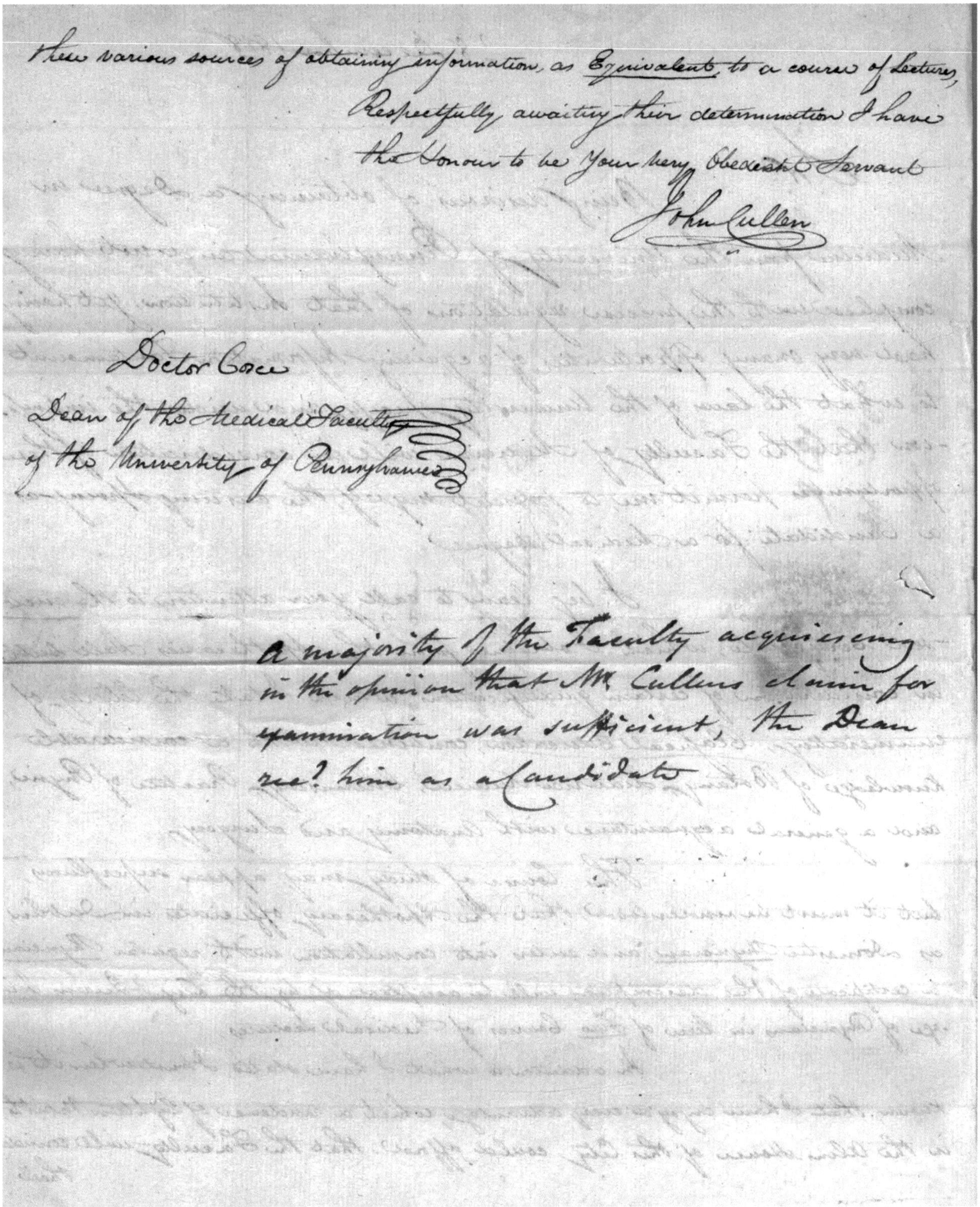
these various sources of obtaining information, as Equivalent to a course of Lectures,
Respectfully awaiting their determination I have
the Honour to be Your very Obedient Servant
John Cullen

Doctor Coxe
Dean of the Medical Faculty
of the University of Pennsylvania

A majority of the Faculty acquiescing
in the opinion that Mr Cullens claim for
examination was sufficient, the Dean
rec'd him as a Candidate

Page 2: John Cullen's handwritten letter December 28, 1818
Request for Accelerated Medical Degree from U of P & Alms House statement
(From the Collections of the University of Pennsylvania Archives)

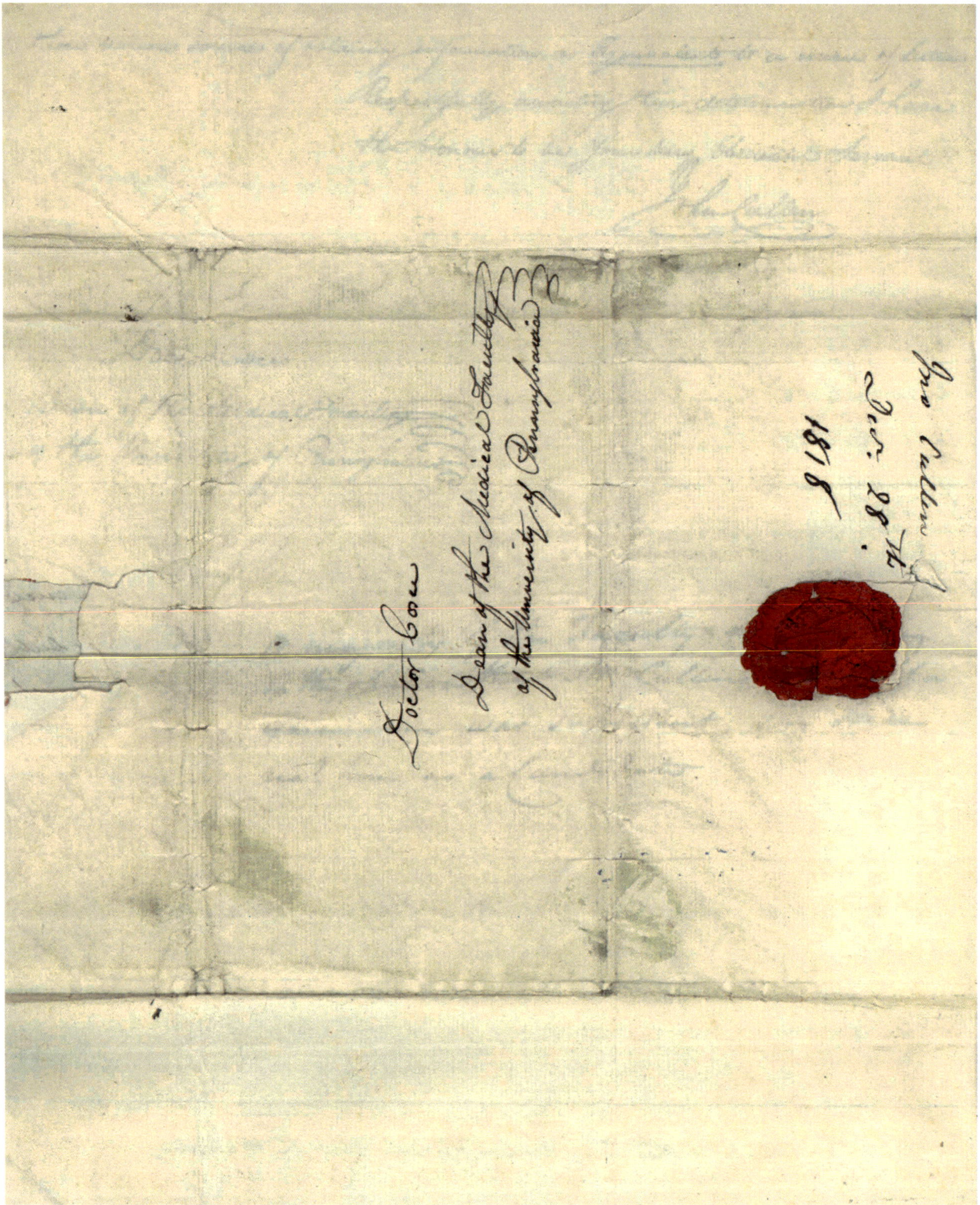

Address Envelope Page to John Cullen's handwritten letter December 28, 1818
Addressed to Dr. Coxe, Dean of the Medical Faculty of University of Pennsylvania
(From the Collections of the University of Pennsylvania Archives)
(Note: Dr John Redman Coxe is the subject of my next volume – Volume 2)

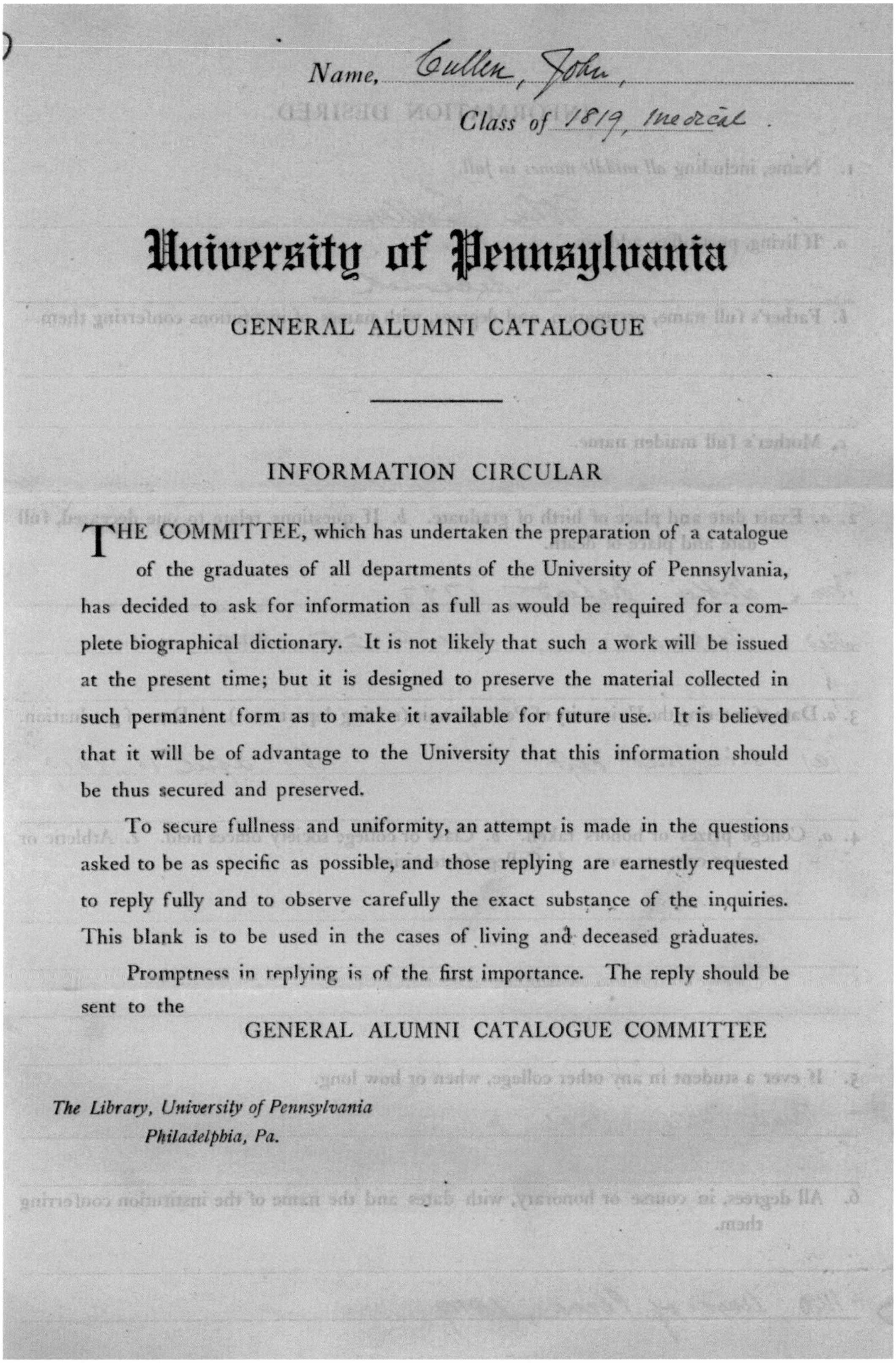

Name, Cullen, John,

Class of 1819, medical.

University of Pennsylvania

GENERAL ALUMNI CATALOGUE

INFORMATION CIRCULAR

THE COMMITTEE, which has undertaken the preparation of a catalogue of the graduates of all departments of the University of Pennsylvania, has decided to ask for information as full as would be required for a complete biographical dictionary. It is not likely that such a work will be issued at the present time; but it is designed to preserve the material collected in such permanent form as to make it available for future use. It is believed that it will be of advantage to the University that this information should be thus secured and preserved.

To secure fullness and uniformity, an attempt is made in the questions asked to be as specific as possible, and those replying are earnestly requested to reply fully and to observe carefully the exact substance of the inquiries. This blank is to be used in the cases of living and deceased graduates.

Promptness in replying is of the first importance. The reply should be sent to the

GENERAL ALUMNI CATALOGUE COMMITTEE

The Library, University of Pennsylvania
Philadelphia, Pa.

Page1: John Cullen Alumni record – University of Pennsylvania
(From the Collections of the University of Pennsylvania Archives)

INFORMATION DESIRED

1. Name, including *all middle names in full*.

John Cullen

a. If living, post-office address.

– deceased –

b. Father's full name, occupation, and degrees, with names of institutions conferring them.

c. Mother's full maiden name.

2. *a*. Exact date and place of birth of graduate. *b*. If questions relate to one deceased, full date and place of death.

Born = Dublin, Ireland, 1797.

Died = Richmond, Va., December 25, 1849.

3. *a*. Date of entering the University of Pennsylvania (stating department). *b*. Date of graduation.

(a) 1816. Med^l dept. (b) April 15, 1819.

4. *a*. College prizes or honors taken. *b*. Class or college society offices held. *c*. Athletic or other contests won. *d*. College fraternities.

5. If ever a student in any other college, when or how long.

Trinity College, Dublin, Ir.

6. All degrees, in course or honorary, with dates and the name of the institution conferring them.

M.D., Univ. of Penna., 1819.

Page2: John Cullen Alumni record – University of Pennsylvania
(From the Collections of the University of Pennsylvania Archives)

7. Occupation since leaving the University. Positions held (business, professional or honorary), with dates wherever possible.

Physician - Studied in Paris, 1814-16.
One of the founders of the Medical College of
Virginia in 1838.

8. Learned societies of which a member.

9. List of publications or original researches made. (For additional titles, see separate sheet.)

10. If ever engaged in military or naval service, state what, when, and where, with rank held, and any important facts. Give dates where possible.

11. If married, give (*a*) date of marriage, (*b*) full maiden name of wife and (*c*) name of wife's father, with his occupation and academic degrees, if any.

Married - Miss Howard of Va.

12. Full names of all children. (State, if none.)

13. Names of relatives among the alumni and degree of relationship.

Place opposite name of relative, name of person to whom application may be made for information respecting him.

It will aid the completion of our record if you will give:

A. Any information respecting deceased alumni and the names of those to whom application may be made.

B. References to any printed biographical matter respecting the alumni, whether living or dead.

Name and full post-office address of person answering the questions.

Page3: John Cullen Alumni record – University of Pennsylvania
(From the Collections of the University of Pennsylvania Archives)

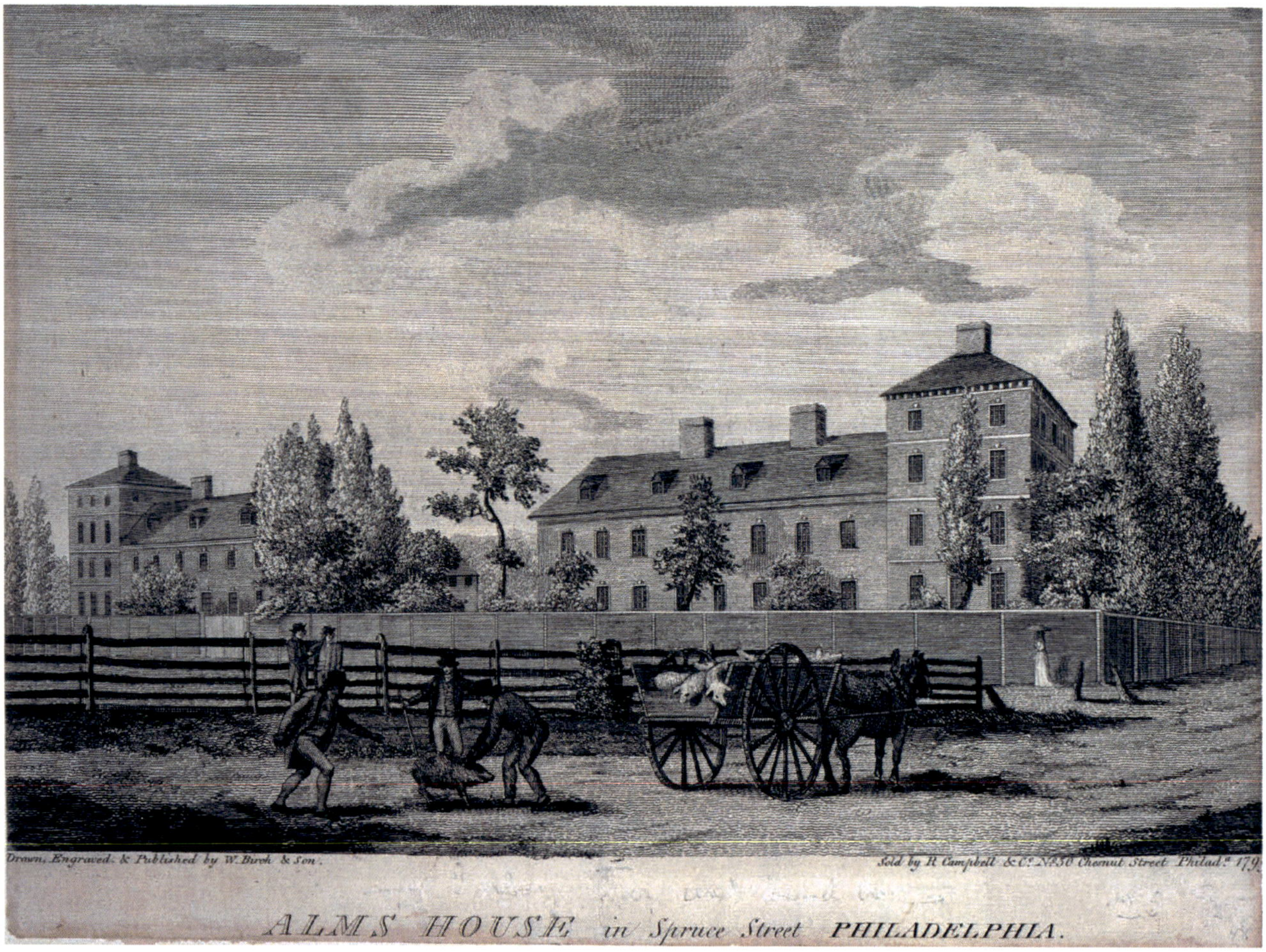

- Philadelphia's Alms House pictured here in 1799 on Spruce Street. John Cullen worked there from June 1817 through December 28, 1818. He may also have been one of the house physicians after obtaining his MD degree in April 1819. This connection may have lasted for another year, until he moved to Richmond Virginia around 1821 or 1822. *Courtesy of "The Library Company of Philadelphia".*

  (Call Number SN 25 / P.2276.59)

- In 1831 a new Alms House was built on the west bank of the Schuylkill River.

- The 1816 Philadelphia Directory by James Robinson describes the Almshouse as an "Almshouse and House of Employment". Lists its location as Spruce Street between 10th and 11th Streets. Apparently the Almshouse was part of a much larger social picture in Philadelphia. It assisted the living as well. The directory shows many pages of guardians of the poor assigned to every block in Philadelphia. It shows two lists of Physicians – one group serving in the Almshouse and another group serving in assigned street locations throughout the city. The magnitude of social support provided the needy in this early time period, is an unexpected surprise.

5.1

Following the Cobblestone Path

The new thread pointing us to Richmond Virginia is very exciting. It is even more compelling because an associated clue mentions that John Cullen is one of the founders of the "Medical College of Virginia" in 1838. It's time for our attention - to move to another region.

We know from the University of Pennsylvania alumni records John Cullen was probably in the Richmond Virginia (area) from 1838 until he passed away in 1849.

However, not so fast, your author has dug other artifacts in Philadelphia with the "Cullen" name on them. From archaeological context and historical documents, I know those artifacts date somewhere between 1847 and 1852. If our "Cullen" is the same one, what is he doing in Philadelphia shortly before passing away in 1849? Historically his "*patent*" was lost in the 1836 fire in Washington and was expired as well (17 year grant of protection 1818 - 1835). Even if Cullen's "*patent*" were still valid, after the 1836 patent office fire, the United States Congress revoked all Patent rights granted to the un-numbered patent holders (X patents) - unless the patents were reconstructed. In communication with the present patent office in Washington D.C. (2006), it has been confirmed Cullen's "*patent*" was never reconstructed. Nothing is known about it.

The other Cullen artifacts are not rare, but definitely scarce and prized when found. Each is a rectangular open pontilled medicine bottle with raised lettering in three of four indented panels stating: "*Rowand and Walton / Philada*" in the front panel, "*Cullen's*" in one of the side panels, and "*Remedies*" in the other side panel. They are aqua in color. Historical records show this partnership were druggists in Philadelphia in the period 1848 through 1851, (although each partner existed independently before and after this date range). Any relationship to John Cullen remains an open question we will revisit later as the clues unfold.

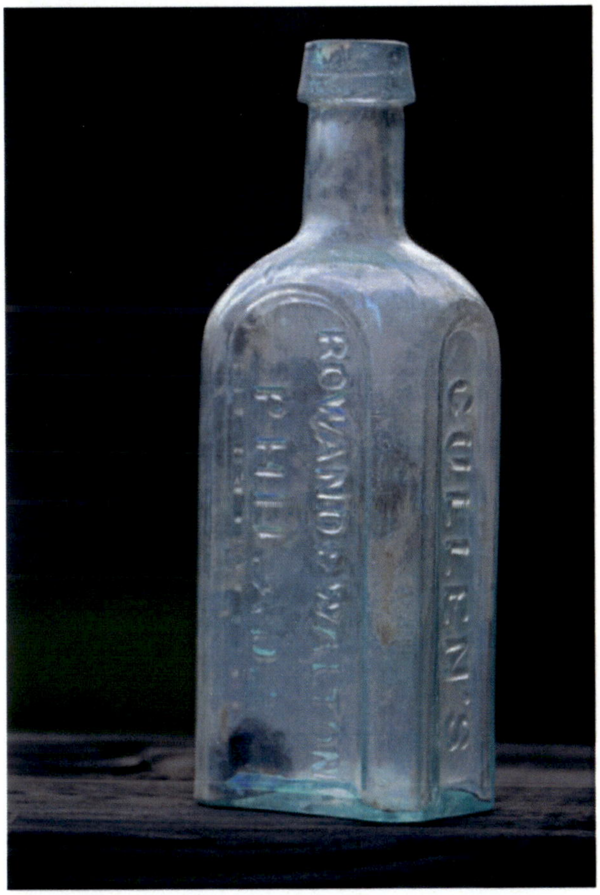

Rowand & Walton / Philada // Cullen's // Remedies, 1848-1851

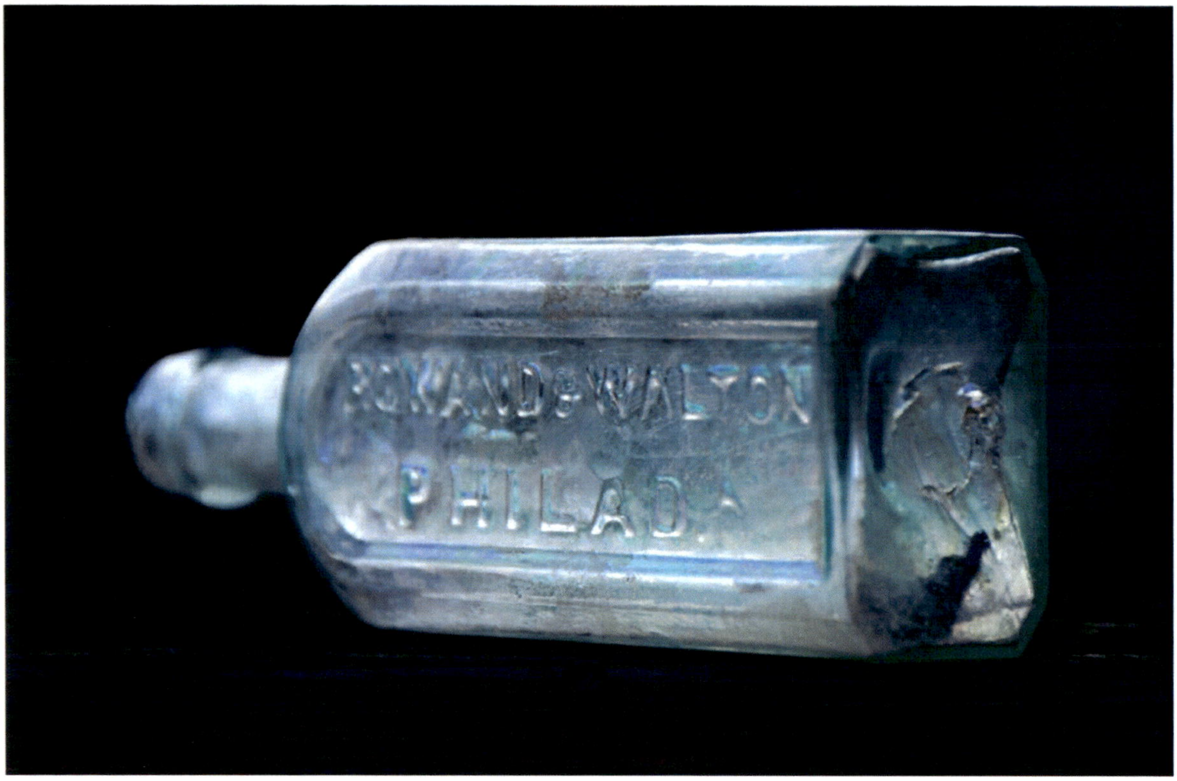

Open pontil base of the "Rowand and Walton" artifact, ("Cullen's" is embossed in top side panel, and "Remedies" embossed in the bottom side panel), 1848-1851.

- ***Can we find any direct historical evidence Cullen was in Virginia from 1822 through 1838?***
- ***What was he doing? Was he practicing Medicine? Was he teaching? Was he a druggist, or performing a combination of these occupations?***

Our new questions may be more difficult because any transition point in a person's life is usually filled with turmoil. Normally the best records in this early period will be city directories. But they are minimal for Richmond Virginia in the 1820's. Even the big microfilm houses have no years between 1819 and 1845. This is not good – perhaps a show stopper – oh well its time for alternatives. Maybe we can locate some ancestry information?

Cullen family records span many volumes. So I decide to use one of my previous clues. John Cullen is originally from Dublin Ireland. But, an internet search of Cullen family records in Ireland is leading nowhere. Still, I continue although I'm not sure what motivated me. Finally an entry that is curious, mentions, a "*medical bill from a John Cullen dated 1824, is attached if anyone is interested*". It must be a different John Cullen because I'm working the Irish family records on a Dublin Ireland internet site? His Irish connection would most likely exist for 1797 through 1816 (the missing period going backward in time from our Alumni document clues). In the year 1824 John Cullen was more likely living in Virginia rather than Ireland (according to hints in our Alumni document). However, I open the internet record and the word "Richmond jumps out of the terminal at me. I can hardly believe it! The coincidence is just incredible.

The medical bill is handwritten and addressed to "*The Proprietor of Negro Woman Dicey*". The handwriting matches the handwriting in the letter from the University of Pennsylvania and, most importantly, the signature of John Cullen is a perfect duplicate. Wow!

The bill is dated "1824" and the location is specified as "Richmond". *So our character is living in Virginia from 1824 through 1849 according to direct historical evidence.* Apparently, for some unknown reason John Cullen left Philadelphia around 1821 or 1822 and appears to be practicing medicine as a Doctor in Richmond Virginia. I can't help wondering if John Cullen felt uncomfortable dealing with slavery issues since he clearly emigrated from parts of the world where his exposure to slavery was minimal or not at all? Further, the bill shows he bled the patient – a practice that was beginning to change at that time (1824). Was he clinging to medical practices that were not progressive – surely University of Pennsylvania was progressive enough to have largely abandoned such extreme measures of dubious medical value? Perhaps my initial reaction is wrong – I may be corrected later when error analysis exposes the answer.

We need to continue following our trail of crumbs. The Alumni records also mention John Cullen founded the Medical College of Virginia in 1838. The historical records lead us to Richmond so I suspect this college must be in the area also. After some investigation, I locate a large university in Richmond called "*Virginia Commonwealth University*" that has a medical school as part of it. The internet discloses a number of libraries. This is normal as mentioned before – so let's decide to skip the main library and search out the telephone number for the Medical library.

Calling the reference desk number, a helpful librarian answers and I ask if he has ever heard of the "*Medical College of Virginia*". He answers "Yes"! He says it has had various names over the years. He lists them for me culminating in his current college name (VCU). This is great news -Terrific! I ask if he knows who the founders were and is one of them named John Cullen? Yes, he responds. I ask if he has any pictures or written material about him or written by him? Yes! He promises to gather up some preliminary material and forward it to me.

A few hours later I'm on cloud nine! The materials arrive and it's our character. A picture of his Richmond, Virginia house and portrait is enclosed. Biographical information written in the 1800's by colleagues, former students, patients, and peers is enclosed. This feels very personal now - as if we have come to know John Cullen.

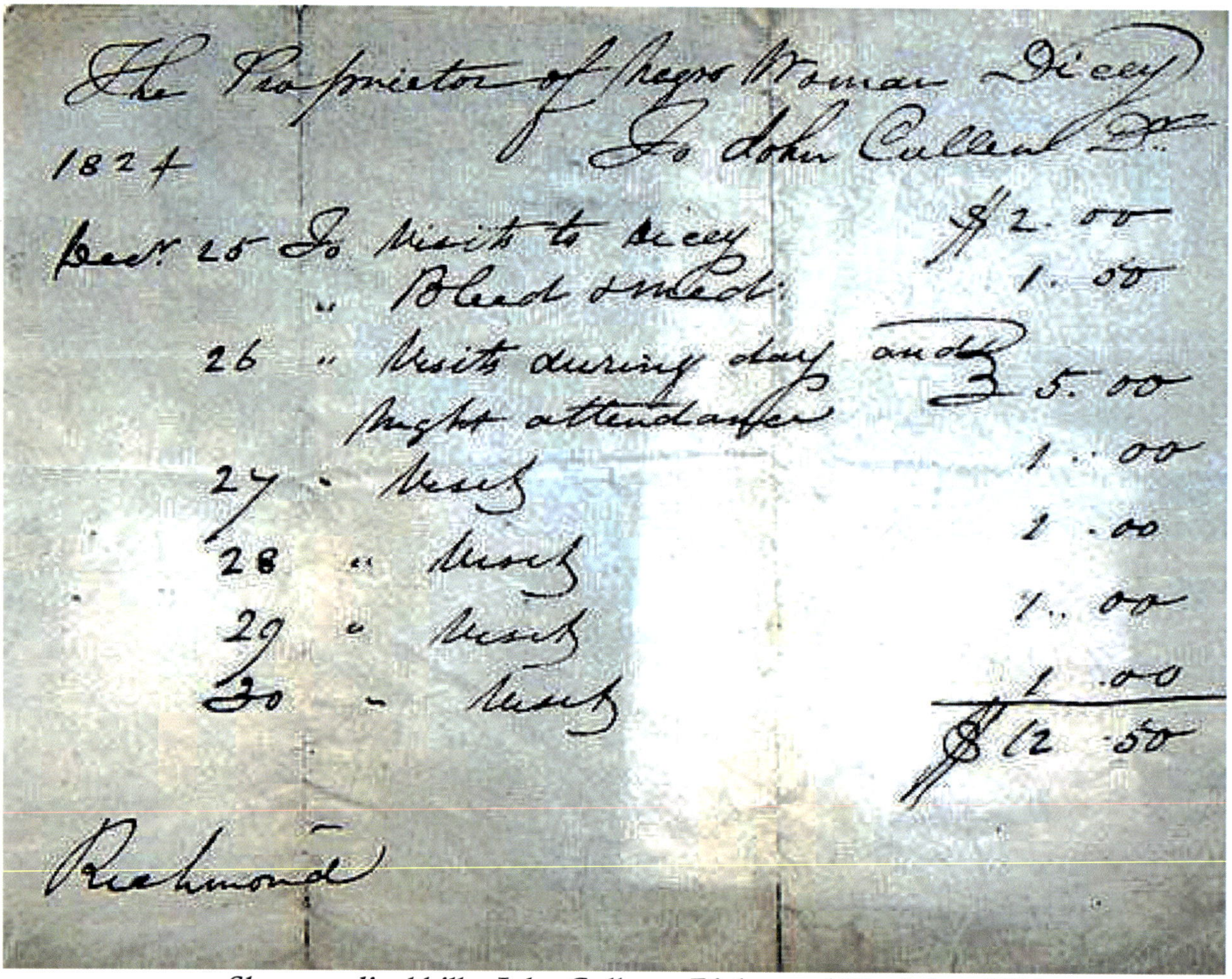

The Proprietor of Negro Woman Dicey
To John Cullen Dr.

1824

Decr. 25	To	Visits to Dicey	$2.00
	"	Bleed & med:	1.00
26	"	Visits during day and night attendance	5.00
27	"	Visit	1.00
28	"	Visit	1.00
29	"	Visit	1.00
30	"	Visit	1.00
			$12.00

Richmond

Slave medical bill – John Cullen – Richmond Virginia – 1824

Dr. John Cullen (1797-1849) - medical bill dated 1824 in Richmond (Virginia) and made out to "The Proprietor of Negro Woman Dicey", Courtesy Alex Peck – Antique Scientifica

The records from VCU disclose that John Cullen was a full professor at "*Medical College of Virginia*" (MCV), from its founding in 1838 until his death in 1849. The biographical materials say he received his medical degree from "*University of Pennsylvania*" (further confirming his Philadelphia roots). Also mentioning he practiced as a physician in Richmond with a large following. The MCV 125th Anniversary edition of the alumni newsletter, "*Medicovan*", March 1962, (p.8.), claims John Cullen married Charlotte Howard of England in 1827, although references to marriage records of Richmond, Virginia list the date as February 28, 1828. Both sources are unreliable because they are not OSD sources - See "*Dodd, Jordan, Research*", Bountiful, Utah – Early American Marriages, Virginia 1740 to 1850. Further research is needed to confirm if either is correct.

They had four children – two sons and two daughters. The eldest son was named after a famous Philadelphia surgeon, "*John Syng Dorsey*". This son eventually became dean of the MCV in 1885 and was also a physician. MCV was merged with other Richmond colleges to form the larger university known today as "*Virginia Commonwealth University*", (VCU) in Richmond.

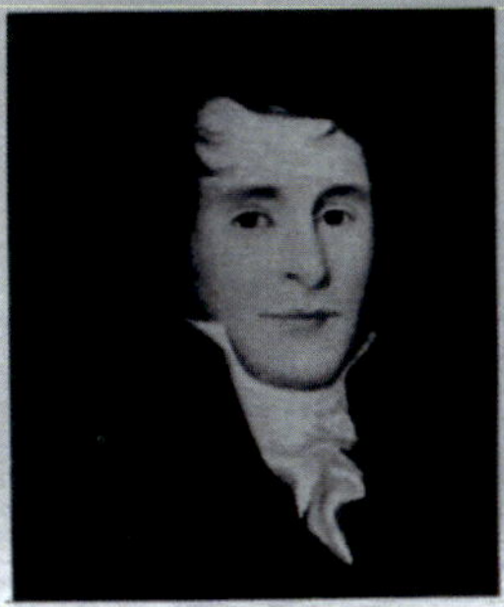

DR. RICHARD LAFON BOHANNAN
1790-1855
Professor of Obstetrics and Diseases of Women and Children

Son of Colonel Joseph Bohannan and Elizabeth Lafon Bohannan. His father was a Captain in the Revolutionary War, and his mother the daughter of Colonel Richard Lafon of the French troops under General Lafayette.

Doctor Bohannan at 48 married a girl of 16. Elizabeth, one of his six children, was a beloved teacher in the South Richmond schools for twenty-five years.

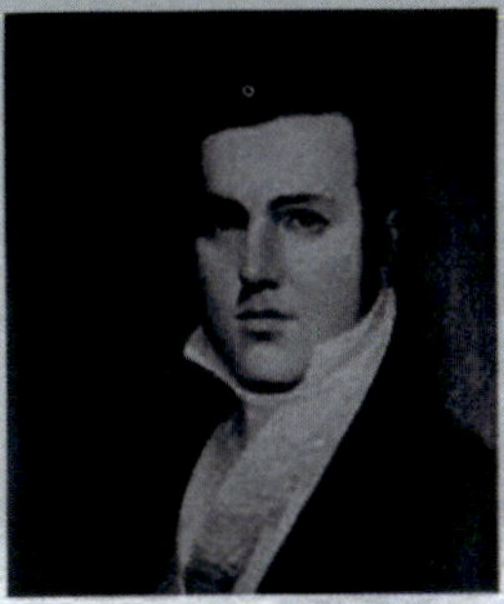

DR. JOHN CULLEN
1797-1849
Professor of Theory and Practice of Medicine

Perhaps the most colorful of the founders, John Cullen, was from Dublin, Ireland. "He was a fine specimen of manhood. Everyone who saw him was struck with his splendid physique. His stature was large, full six feet tall, his person round, his face full with rosy cheeks, with every capillary filled with florid blood, his eye, a large laughing blue one, his hair light brown and disposed to curl." (Dr. T. Pollard)

He had a reputation as an orator. It was said that "he can suit in voice, language, and manner the roughest Son of the Brogue, or the most courtly and polished gentleman."

In 1827, he married Charlotte Howard of England. They had two sons and two daughters. One son, Dr. John Syng Dorsey Cullen, became professor of surgery and dean of MCV in 1885.

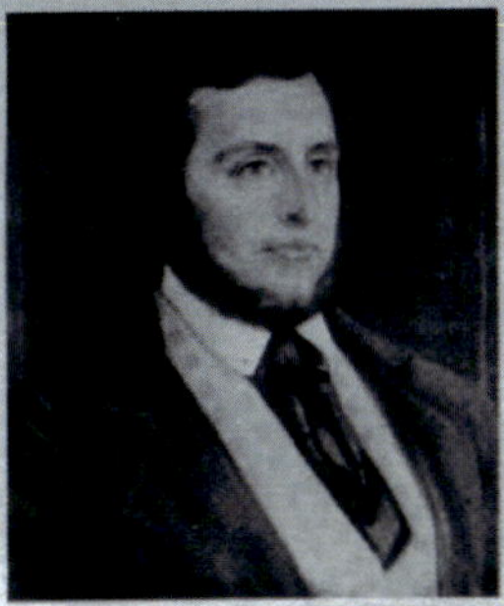

DR. AUGUSTUS LOCKMAN WARNER
1807-1847
Dean and Professor of Surgery and Surgical Anatomy

Doctor Warner is described by Dr. L. B. Anderson as "of medium stature, exceedingly handsome face, brilliant blue eyes, a soft musical voice, easy and graceful manners, and great fluency of speech."

We read in the **Richmond Times and Compiler** July 11, 1845, that he operated on the lower jaw of a patient exposing a 13" tumor, and removed it and two-thirds of the jaw in 9 minutes. After the operation, the patient walked from the room.

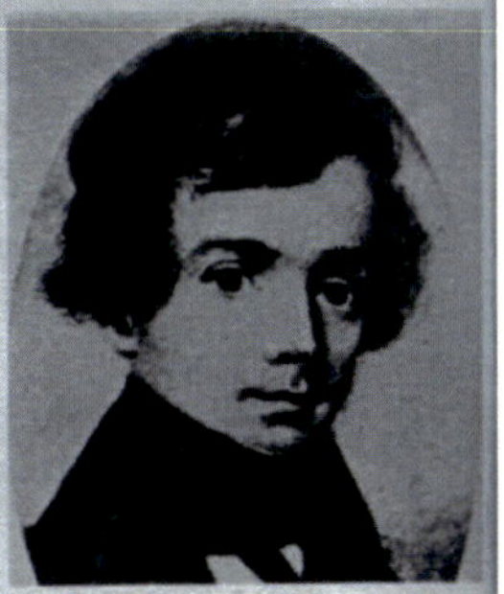

DR. ROBERT MUNFORD
1816-1843
Demonstrator of Anatomy

Dr. Robert Munford, the first demonstrator of anatomy, (not considered a "faculty position" in the rules and regulations; so he is not considered one of the founders) was the son of William and Sarah Radford Munford. He attended the University of Virginia for one session, 1834-35. In 1838, he married Anne Elizabeth Curtis, who was the daughter of Dr. Henry Curtis and Christiana Tyler Curtis of Hanover County, the latter a sister of President John Tyler. Mrs. Anne Curtis Munford lived until 1917, her ninety-seventh year.

From 1850 to 1869 she conducted a school in the basement of the William Munford House at Canal and Fifth streets. General William Gorgas, hero of the yellow fever fight in the Panama Canal Zone, was a pupil here and known as "little Willie Gorgas."

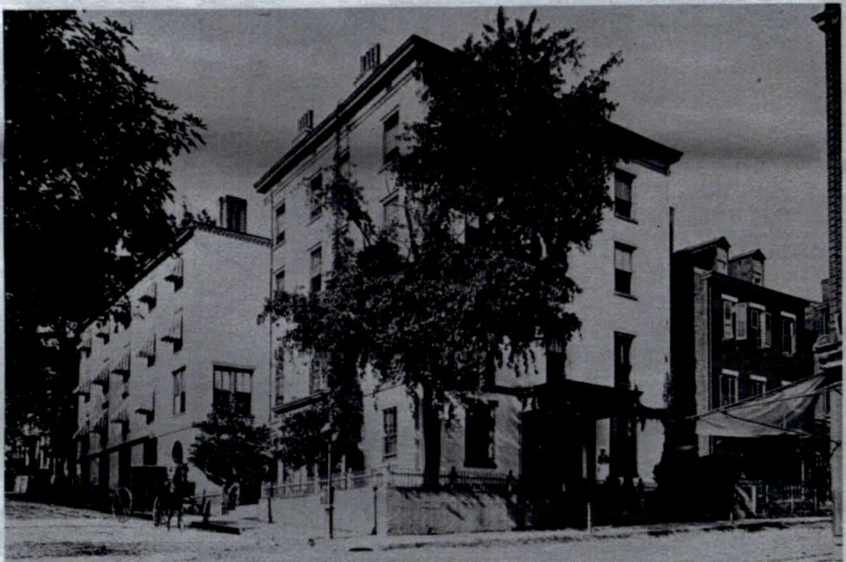

HOME OF DOCTOR CULLEN on the corner of Ross and Governor Streets "with commodious offices on the first floor." It was here the original Saint Luke's Hospital was opened in 1883.

This page is from the "Bulletin of the Medical College of Virginia vol. 61, No.1, Page 6, "The first 125 Years of the Medical College of Virginia", published Fall 1963 – John Cullen is pictured second from left and his home is pictured below it - *Courtesy of "Special Collections and Archives, Thompkins - McCaw Library, Virginia Commonwealth University.*

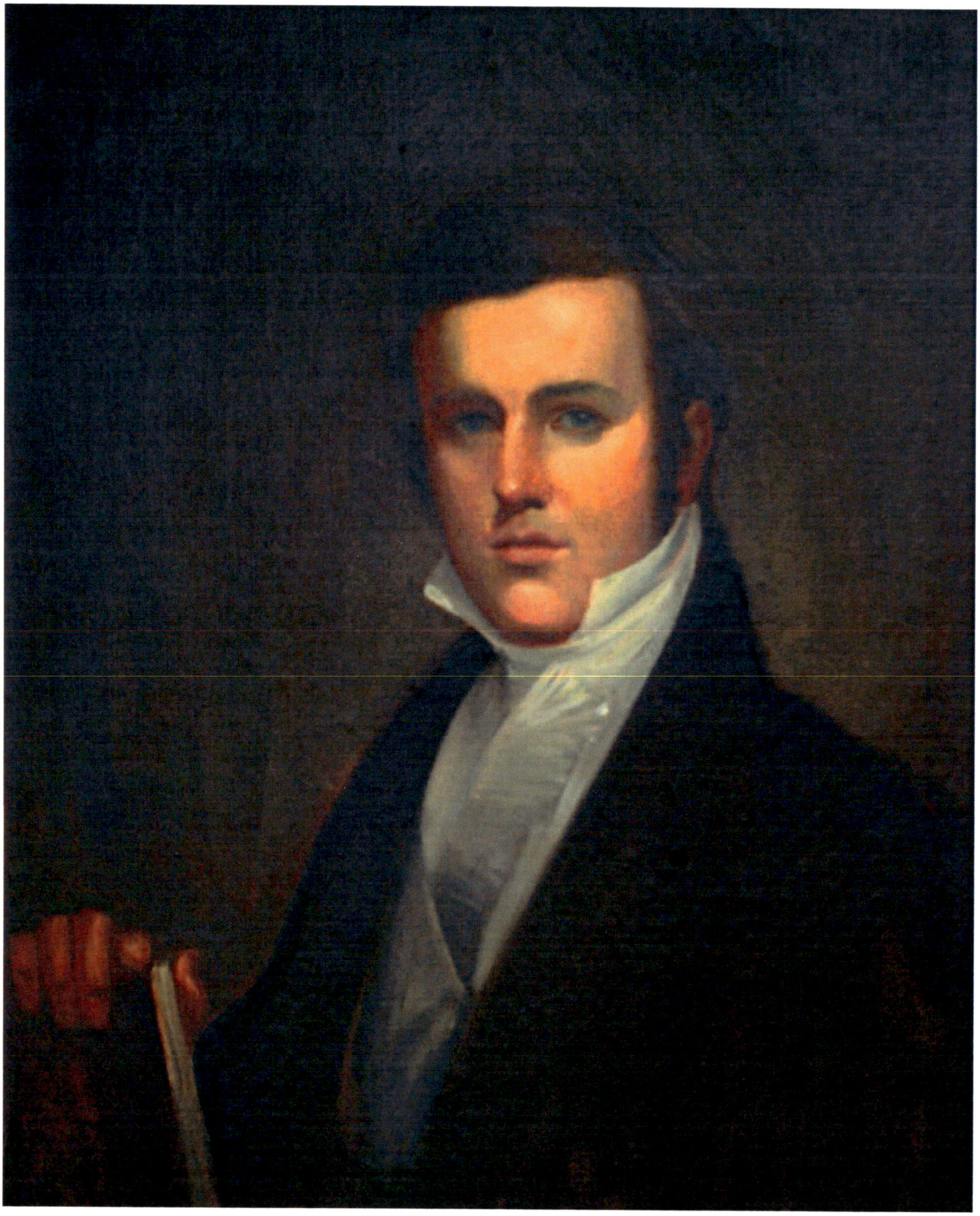

John Cullen portrait (oil on Canvas), photograph by Clement Strudwick.
Courtesy of "Special Collections and Archives, Thompkins - McCaw Library, Virginia Commonwealth University.

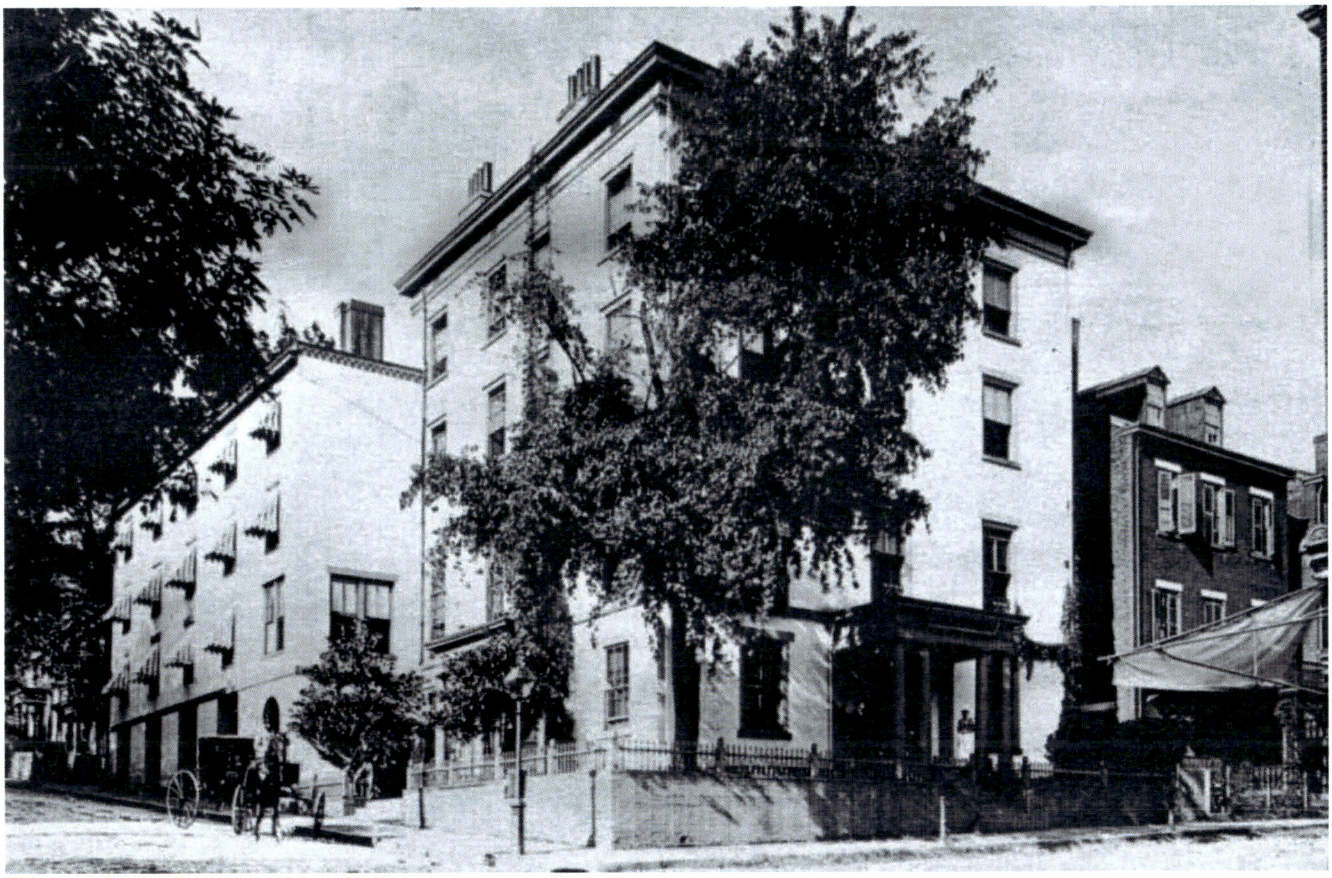

Photograph of John Cullen's residence as St. Luke's Hospital, Richmond, Virginia. *Courtesy of "Special Collections and Archives, Thompkins - McCaw Library, Virginia Commonwealth University.*

The records from VCU confirm that Doctor Cullen traveled to Philadelphia in 1849. His purpose was to obtain help for a serious illness. He may have made other trips in 1847/48 for much the same reason, although there is no evidence of this. He probably had a progressive illness and knew, as it became worse, that his affairs needed to be resolved. I suspect, knowing he was ill, and having business affairs left behind from his previous years in Philadelphia, he made agreements that resulted in the introduction of his remedies by "*Rowand and Walton*" around 1848 or 1849. The directory entries in Philadelphia appear to support this theory (as does the archaeological record). The only years when "*Rowand and Walton*" is listed as a partnership are those in the chart below. Cullen's remedies had an abrupt and short duration (1848/49 – 1851). There is no evidence Cullen's remedies were continued after the "*Rowand and Walton*" partnership dissolved.

Year	Listed Name	Philadelphia Address	Occupation	Ref
1848	Rowand & Walton	376 High St.	Druggists	1
1849	Rowand & Walton	376 High St.	Druggists	1
1850	Rowand & Walton	21 N 6th St.	Druggists	1
1851	Rowand & Walton	21 N 6th St.	Druggists	1

Most importantly the clues now fill our character with the vibrancy and exhilaration of his times. By way of illustration, the biographical material from VCU reveals *John Cullen* was briefly affected by two of the most significant names in world history, whose reputations thunder down through the ages to us. Few individuals ascend to such historical levels as *Thomas Jefferson* and *Napoleon Bonaparte*. How John Cullen came to be touched by these two legends is a marvelous story.

Although John Cullen's life is changed by both Jefferson and Napoleon, it was as if each tale had occurred on a separate planet. The events were so isolated in time and place that we have two separate stories with threads swirling off in all directions.

A short biography was written by Dr. T. Pollard of Richmond Virginia, who claims to have personally known John Cullen as a patient and as a hospital student. These memoirs were set forth in the *Atlantic Journal of Medicine*, entitled "*Sketch of the Life of Dr. John Cullen." Atlantic Journal of Medicine, v.1, no. 3 (October 1883), pages 191-199).* This OSD confirms many of the preceding answers as well as details of John Cullen's everyday life after leaving Philadelphia. It is less detailed about his time before coming to Philadelphia.

Details of his time in Philadelphia are mixed up and contain significant errors, as I document following the large quotation below.

Let's begin with Napoleon. In the biography, Dr. Pollard writes:

"About 1814 he (John Cullen) visited Paris, with a view of further prosecuting his studies, and from this city, by invitation, he started to visit his uncle, Bishop Curtis, of the Catholic Church, Salamanca, Spain. Bishop Curtis, on account of his kindness to the sick and wounded in Wellington's army in the Peninsula campaign, won the gratitude and favor of that distinguished General, who through his influence with the Pope afterwards secured for him the high position of Primate of Ireland. On his way to Spain, Dr. Cullen was arrested by the French authorities, as an English subject, in accordance with Napoleon's order, following the Berlin and Milan decrees, and was carried to Paris as a prisoner. He was paroled and allowed to go at large, and then resumed his studies, acquiring a knowledge of the French language and prosecuting studies in anatomy and operative surgery. During his stay in Paris, of one or two years, he made the acquaintance of many of the distinguished men of that capital – men prominent in science, politics and art, and gained an entre to the salons of the wits and savants of the gay city. It may have been here that he acquired the taste for wit and satire, which afterwards distinguished him, or it may have been a school to him to develop and educate a natural taste in that direction. While in Paris, he at one time, became the guest of the distinguished poet Chateaubriand. After the battle of Waterloo, Dr. Cullen returned to England, in the same ship with the "Allied Sovereigns", on their visit to that country." *(continued on page 52)*

Since this is second hand information, I caution the reader, it should be viewed in a general light rather than specific. Memories are faded and much of the detail was likely forgotten or mixed up by the 1880's when this was written. If John Cullen had compiled a diary or biography while he was living, a clearer picture might emerge. Perhaps further investigation can locate first person documents (by John Cullen or institutional records) to corroborate or contradict the biographical material.

What we know for certain is, "Coalition Forces" under the Duke of Wellington and German Field-Marshal Blucher defeated Napoleon at Waterloo (Belgium near Brussels) on June 18, 1815. Napoleon escaped capture for awhile, surrendering on July 15, 1815 to British Navy Captain Maitland of the "*Bellerophon*".

The "*Allied Sovereign*" monarchs and Louis XVIII arrived in Paris around July 7, 1815. Of course the coalition Armies were occupying Paris at that time as well. The English sent Napoleon to the island of St. Helena where he died on May 5, 1821.

John Cullen returned to England with the "*Allied Sovereign*" leaders sometime shortly after July 7, 1815. Discovering the exact date John Cullen arrived in America is a tale in itself and follows on the next several pages. This closed the European chapter of his life. Although he later married an English woman (1827/28, in Virginia) it is not likely he returned because his biographers claim he never took a vacation.

The tales he must have known in this storied period of time. To be on the scene of the action and power, in Paris, – spending time as a prisoner of Napoleon and then paroled – perhaps seeing Napoleon himself during his return to power in the legendary 100 days. Knowing many of the insiders and famous, he certainly would have had the opportunity. All this before he ever arrives in Philadelphia. Fantastic!

After Dr. Cullen's time in France, came his experiences in Philadelphia. The period of time from late 1815 through early 1816, when John Cullen likely immigrated to Philadelphia, was absolutely confirmed by following a series of obscure clues which lead me to a wonderful OSD from October 28th, 1817. Even the thinnest of threads can open a window otherwise lost in the mists of time. These clues by themselves are so weak that they are nothing but a series of comical errors in the shadows. A rare book from 1816 is the clue. The book's subject would suggest a determination to become an American citizen. In theory the book was used by John Cullen in 1816 or 1817. Although based on very thin evidence mentioned below, ultimately it leads to a fabulous find. The theory is that: In 1816 John Cullen purchased the book titled "*An essay on Naturalization and Allegiance…*" by *John F DuMoulin*, and (*published by Daniel Rapine, Washington City, 1816*). The title suggesting John Cullen is studying to become an American and wishes to succeed in his new homeland. The year of publication just happens to be the same year, (1816), that we speculate John immigrated to the US (based on the sketchy biography material of Dr. T. Pollard and the alumni records from the University of Pennsylvania).

In theory, why did I believe this book was used by John Cullen? Because it appeared John may have left a wonderful clue that had silently sailed the generations for me to find. Through an extremely odd series of coincidences, the Huntingdon Library in California made a series of mistakes while "*copy cataloging*" their own copy of the same book (not actually having been owned or possessed by John Cullen). They accidentally copied part of the catalog entry from another library which happened to include a strange reference to someone named John Cullen. Unfortunately the Huntingdon Library was unable to reconstruct the source of the original catalog entry. So we cannot locate and print for you what follows in the next paragraph.

According to the "*copied catalog*" entry someone named John Cullen repeatedly signed his name on the front endpaper of the book - over and over again, as if practicing as a school child would when first learning to write. This mistaken catalog entry resided in the Huntington Research Library in San Marino, California, "*Eames Collection, Call No. 190835*". Based on my query they have now fixed their mistake but oddly the one person who likely would recognize and follow the immigration clue, myself, found it, and realized its significance. Research is often about these strange twists of fate. Science is full of great discoveries made after a mistake, or accident, or series of errors. In this case it leads me to yet another spectacular historical connection of the greatest rarity, that no one understood or realized – including the Huntington Library.

The question raised by the mistaken Huntington Library record, is as follows.

Is there any immigration OSD evidence corroborating that John Cullen actually applied for or became a United States citizen in 1816 or 1817?

Keep in mind, that in the early period of US history, local courts often recorded declarations of citizenship and "oaths of allegiance".

So what court in Philadelphia may have done so? Do records exist?

I suspect a little known Philadelphia department that I've used a few times may hold these records. It is called the "*Philadelphia City Archives*" which holds some records from the "*Mayor's Court*" from the early 1800's. After a brief trip to the archives a terrific discovery is made: Yes, naturalization records show John Cullen declared allegiance October 28, 1817, wishing to become a naturalized American citizen, *(Ref: Microfilm roll # 21.17 (964556) from 1814 – 1838 of the court's Naturalization Docket, as well as, the actual document as identified in the "Descriptive Inventory of Archives of the City & County of Philadelphia" by John Daly (1970)- Mayor's Court docket # 130.3 – 7 Volumes – Item 57 of the Naturalization Docket (1814 - 1838.)*

The court record shows John declared he migrated from Dublin, Ireland, arriving in New York, September 29, 1815, confirming my earlier speculation as to when John left Paris and immigrated to the United States.

All of the written material appears to be in John Cullen's distinctive flowing script. The signature at the bottom is a match to his letter of December 28, 1818 written to the *University of Pennsylvania medical college* – (*see page 33*). So, again we have clear historical evidence from an OSD source about John Cullen – no guessing and no hearsay. He gives his date of birth as February 2nd, 1796 and claims he is 21 years old in 1817. States he was born in the County of Dublin, in Ireland and was born a member of the British Nation, owing allegiance to the King of the United Kingdom of Great Britain and Ireland.

He further states that it is his intention to settle in the City of Philadelphia. This is fabulous evidence of John's status at this key point in time with no biographical mistakes clouding our tale.

From previous OSD sources we know John Cullen has been attending the University Of Pennsylvania Medical College since 1816, as well as starting his druggist business on Chestnut Street during the year of 1817. Also, from his letter to the Medical College December 28th. 1818 we know John has been working (or volunteering) at the Philadelphia Alms House on Spruce Street since June 1817. So his time in New York was about one year - more or less.

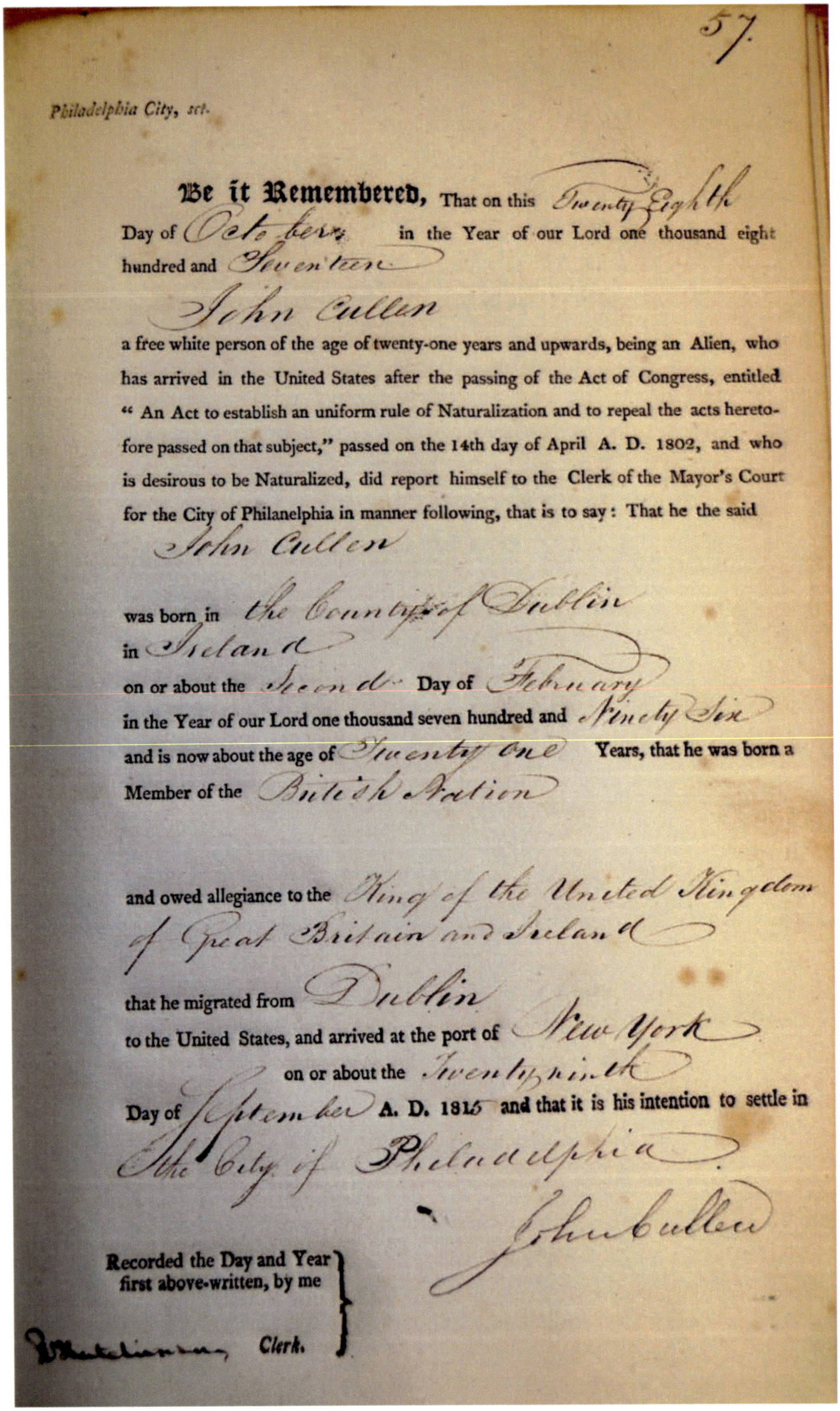

57

Philadelphia City, sct.

Be it Remembered, That on this Twenty Eighth Day of October in the Year of our Lord one thousand eight hundred and Seventeen

John Cullen

a free white person of the age of twenty-one years and upwards, being an Alien, who has arrived in the United States after the passing of the Act of Congress, entitled "An Act to establish an uniform rule of Naturalization and to repeal the acts heretofore passed on that subject," passed on the 14th day of April A. D. 1802, and who is desirous to be Naturalized, did report himself to the Clerk of the Mayor's Court for the City of Philanelphia in manner following, that is to say: That he the said John Cullen

was born in the County of Dublin in Ireland on or about the Second Day of February in the Year of our Lord one thousand seven hundred and Ninety Six and is now about the age of Twenty One Years, that he was born a Member of the British Nation

and owed allegiance to the King of the United Kingdom of Great Britain and Ireland

that he migrated from Dublin to the United States, and arrived at the port of New York on or about the Twentyninth Day of September A. D. 1815 and that it is his intention to settle in the City of Philadelphia

John Cullen

Recorded the Day and Year first above-written, by me

[illegible] Clerk.

John Cullen's immigration declaration – Philadelphia Mayor's Court October 28th, 1817 - *City of Philadelphia, Department of Records, City Archives*

Because I believed the Huntington Library's catalog was correct when I first checked - before their mistake was unraveled – I was hopeful of discovering other possible documents related to John Cullen in their archives. So, I queried other Huntington Library departments by telephone. To my amazement I uncover many more OSD documents relating to John Cullen that their online catalogs did not itemize or list. I had not expected to find this much new information in California so far removed from Philadelphia. I should mention, the absence of manuscripts in a catalog is not unusual (letters and personal documents). They are generally not in open catalogs and it is always important to dig a little deeper. Persistence will be rewarded.

In this case I discover many other personal letters of Dr. Cullen's family in the Huntington Library. The letters are salacious in content and date from the 1840's relating to John's relationship with his wife. At the end of this chapter, an interesting examination evolves.

Getting back to Dr T. Pollard's biographical material, I can document a number of omissions and mix-ups within this material as it pertains to Cullen's time from 1816 through 1821 (in Philadelphia). These prompted my caution to you, several pages previous, about blindly accepting "*second hand information*" - illustrating the dangers of reference quoting and "*the perpetuation of errors*". A few additions and corrections are listed below to illustrate how the biographical material (second hand information) can be mistaken, incomplete, or mixed up:

These facts pertain to the 1815 through 1821 time period and are based on "original source documents", OSD, *(John Cullen's handwritten letter; the marked Cullen artifact; patent index records; "Aurora" Philadelphia newspaper advertisements; Philadelphia directories and their entries; Philadelphia Mayor's Court "Naturalization" records;, John Cullen's personal books; University of Pennsylvania alumni records; etc.)*

OSD Fact: John Cullen worked for himself in his own chemical, druggist, and mineral water (fountain & bottling) business in Philadelphia on Chestnut Street from late 1817 through 1819.

OSD Fact: John Cullen entered the University of Pennsylvania medical school in 1816 and graduated on April 15, 1819.

OSD Fact: John Cullen declared allegiance to the United States of America in Philadelphia October 28, 1817, wishing to become a "Naturalized American" citizen, in "*Philadelphia's Mayor's Court*" and claims he migrated from Dublin Ireland arriving in New York September 29, 1815. States he was born in Dublin on February 2nd, 1796, is 21 years old, and intends to settle in the City of Philadelphia.

OSD Fact: John Cullen worked in the Philadelphia Almshouse from June 1817 through December 28, 1818. (*He may have continued working there after getting his medical degree if Dr. Pollard's biographical information is correct*).

OSD Fact: John Cullen was awarded by "Letters Patent of the U States" the first known patent for soda water itself - at the age of 22 on May 4, 1818 in Philadelphia. (He was likely using James S Ewing's newly patented (1817), explosion proof mineral water manufacturing equipment that made loading of light weight glass bottles possible on a commercial basis.)

Keep in mind some of Dr. Pollard's biographical material below is incomplete or not specifically confirmed by the OSD historical record but is generally correct.

In the biography he writes:

(continued from page 47) *"...A short time afterwards he sailed for New York, where his services, as a chemist, were soon secured by a large manufacturing company, which required the highest attainments in chemistry for the successful prosecution of its business. Remaining in this position for sometime, he then determined to go to Philadelphia, the seat of the most prominent medical school, at that time, in the United States, to complete his medical education. He there became acquainted with Dr. Physick and Dr. Jno.Syng Dorsey, the latter of whom took him, as his private pupil, and gave him full advantages of his operations and dissections. A strong attachment grew up between them, and but for Dr. Dorsey's untimely death, it is probable that they would have been associated in practice, of which Dr. Cullen had had some intimations. We suppose that after Dr. Dorsey, was named our Dr. Dorsey Cullen. After graduating in the medical department of the University of Pennsylvania, Dr. Cullen became the resident physician to the "City Almshouse" of Philadelphia, for a year or more, and, at the expiration of his term of service, he came to Virginia, at the solicitation of Mr. Jefferson, to confer with him in reference to some position, in the University of Virginia, which he wished him to accept; but before going to Charlottesville, he visited his friend and countryman, Dr. Robertson, at Petersburg, and was prevailed upon to remain there long enough to deliver a course of lectures on chemistry. After doing so, he visited Richmond en route to Monticello, but was there stricken down with protracted fever and on his recovery, was urged by many friends, he had formed in Richmond, to make that city his permanent residence. Touched by their generous sympathy, during his protracted illness, he determined to yield to their solicitations, and soon offered himself as a candidate for the practice of medicine."*

The untimely death of John Cullen's friend and mentor, *"John Syng Dorsey"*, in November 1818, changed the course of history. For it is shortly afterwards, John Cullen is asking for an accelerated medical degree in his letter of December 28, 1818 to University of Pennsylvania Medical School. The Philadelphia directory for 1819 lists "*Dorsey, Widow of John S. M.D., 189 Mulberry Street*". John Cullen's "*mineral water business and chemical warehouse*" are apparently stopped abruptly - since it is no longer listed in Philadelphia directories. His loyalty and affection for his friend is obvious when over a decade later he names his first son after him (*John Syng Dorsey Cullen*). He receives his M.D. on April 15,

1819 and quickly opened an office at 92 S Front Street, Philadelphia.

Within approximately a year he is contacted by Thomas Jefferson about a position at Jefferson's beloved University of Virginia, Charlottesville Virginia - if Dr. T. Pollard's biographical material is correct.

It must have been a fabulous honor to receive an invitation from Thomas Jefferson, one of our greatest national heroes and 3rd President of the United States (1801–1809). I can hardly imagine the excitement of directly corresponding with a founding father, who was the actual writer of some of our nation's most cherished documents (Declaration of Independence).

Perhaps correspondence from Pres. Thomas Jefferson exists at Jefferson's library (in Monticello or elsewhere) sent to John Cullen or to others discussing John Cullen's future? Good question for another day and lots more crumbs to follow.

The history above, simply takes my breath away! Recall when we started this book, I mentioned, artifacts could lead to long lost tales that could sweep you off your feet! Well here we are.

During his trip to Virginia to see President Jefferson, John Cullen becomes ill and is mended in Richmond Virginia. He was so touched by the kindness received – he decides to stay, open an office, and practice medicine. That John Cullen stayed in Richmond is clear from the medical bill dated 1824, Richmond (Virginia) and made out to "*The Proprietor of Negro Woman Dicey*" bearing the signature of John Cullen. (*See picture displayed in a previous chapter.*)

Dr. Pollard continues the biographical article, stating that after Dr. Cullen became a prominent physician in Richmond (1822 – 1838), that:

> *"In 1838, he, in conjunction with Drs. Bohannon, Warren (Warner), Chamberlayne, Johnston, and Maupin, established the present Medical College of Virginia. To Dr. Cullen was assigned the chair of Practice of medicine. He was equally competent to have filled any other professorship in the institution.*
>
> *The writer's acquaintance with Dr. Cullen commenced in the winter of 1839, as a student in the institution, with which he was connected."*

The founding in 1838, of one of the most famous medical colleges in the United States, (Medical College of Virginia), is a crucial moment in history. Far from Paris and John's Irish heritage, as well as his grief and loss in Philadelphia - he steps up to the plate and hits a home run for all of us that follow in his footsteps. John rises again quietly and heroic, the classic American tale of standing up and making a go of things no matter where you are in life. His lifelong devotion to the Medical College and its success is the long term determination we all admire so much in our heroes. So now we have the rounding out of three separate and distinct periods in John Cullen's life – as if they occurred on separate planets. His family and his college will occupy the rest of his life.

After describing many personal details of Dr. Cullen's lectures, appearance, habits, and interesting antidotes, Dr Pollard writes of his untimely passing:

"Dr. Cullen died 25th December 1849, in the 52nd year of his age, of softening of the brain, induced, in all probability, by the incessant activity of that organ, and his unceasing professional labors. In the thirty years of his practice, he had not allowed himself a single vacation – a commentary on the unwise habit of keeping the "bow always bent". (Nequae Apolle arcum simper tendit.) We remember that he went to Philadelphia, to consult some of the medical faculty, wishing that they would order venesection for him – they did not do so. He returned to Richmond, and insisted upon having himself bled, which was done. Dr. Bohannon told me he had no doubt this treatment hastened his end.

His remains rest in Hollywood, beneath a tall granite monolith, with the simple inscription of the time and place of his birth and death.

Dr. Cullen left two sons, Dr. J. Dorsey Cullen, now professor of Surgery in the Medical College of Virginia, and Matthew Cullen, of St. Louis, where he has held important positions in the city government, and two daughters, Mrs. Col. H.A. Carrington, of Charlotte, and Mrs. Judge Breathed, of Maryland."

More crumbs – the children are as interesting as the father. One trail includes "*General Robert E. Lee and General Longstreet*" in the Civil War. For example: In the battle of the Wilderness in Virginia on May 6th, 1864 *Lieutenant General James Longstreet* was severely wounded *(cervical wound from friendly fire)*. John's son, *John Syng Dorsey Cullen, MD* controlled the hemorrhage, helped evacuate him from the battlefield, and cared for him during convalescence. Longstreet was arguably the finest corps commander on either side during the Civil War.

As stated earlier, the clues have lead to tales now filling our character with the vibrancy and exhilaration of his times. Far beyond anything I could have imagined on that rainy cold night when I found our artifact!

But wait a minute, "*Charlotte Howard Cullen*", John's wife, will bring some reality to our character. As in real life, most of us have tales we are proud of and those we are not - John Cullen is no exception. Although Dr. Cullen appears to be more than a mere mortal, in reality he was human like all of us. Time tends to distort tales involving heroic characters. Now our tale will acquire a more human face.

On December 9th & 10th, 1844, Charlotte Howard Cullen wrote two versions of the same letter to Chancellor Samuel Taylor of the Medical College of Virginia. These letters form part of a collection originally belonging to James Lyons of Richmond Virginia. Some letters in this collection were written by Charlotte Cullen directly to James Lyons. They are located in the "*Brock Collection, Huntington Library, San Marino California*".

She asked for the Chancellor's counsel concerning divorce in her "*distressing situation*". These documents and others in the Huntington Library's collection apparently were saved for Charlotte's side in a potential divorce trial that ultimately did not occur. Keep in mind when considering the information below, 99% was supplied by Charlotte Cullen and her witnesses. Caution should always be used when only one side in a dispute is presented - the tale can be distorted. So with that in mind I will describe the information. It does not mean the information is accurate or inaccurate – or that I believe one way or the other unless I specifically say so.

In these documents Charlotte described a continual series of events, when taken together over a period of 10 years, suggest John was verbally abusive and mean spirited towards her and some of his own children. Of course the usual money issues come up that plague modern marriages. The difference is, that in the 1840's women were not on an equal footing with men and this lead to many injustices. So any divorce trial was an unusual occurrence and not begun lightly – especially by a woman. Men ruled and women were not believed. Therefore the mere fact that this dispute got to the stage it did – with a lawyer taking depositions etc., gives some credibility to Charlotte's claim of abuse.

Charlotte claimed to be considering suicide unless a divorce from John could be granted. She freely admits to contributing to this unstable behavior by taking opium for 8 years. She claimed repeatedly that John accused her of being crazy and name calling, with the usual purpose of hurting her feelings. He apparently suggested she was on the road to becoming a "*strumpet*" by her own desire. Charlotte accused John of refusing marriage "*reconciliation*" for the past "*eight years this fall, without her approbation*", (fall of 1844).

She also claimed a nurse John hired was coming between them, although she stopped short of claiming infidelity. She states John confided personal family matters and powers over the children to this nurse that should have been for her alone. Often the nurse and John drank strong spirits together and Charlotte was uncomfortable with the nurse being around her children in that condition. Alcohol was on their breath and their inebriated condition was frequently evidenced by their demeanor. Her witnesses claim to have personally seen and counseled John about an alcohol problem as early as 1838.

Of course this does not explain how Charlotte could justify her own opium drug use for 8 years, presumably around these same 4 children. It seems to be a bit of a double standard that most good trial lawyers would soon exploit in front of a jury.

She apparently had the support of Dr. Bohannon whom she claimed was her physician and advised her against reconciliation with John. Remember Dr. Bohannon was one of the founders of the "*Medical College of Virginia*" along with others including Dr. John Cullen in 1838. So it could be presumed he knew Dr. Cullen at least 6 years at that time, and was qualified to give Charlotte such advice.

According to Charlotte's letters Dr. Bohannon "*feared for her sanity and safety*" and that is why he advised her against reconciliation. Included in the "*Huntington Library's Brock Collection*" is a fragment of a deposition taken in 1845. It was taken for the divorce case against Dr. Cullen and lists Dr. Bohannon and Reverend Woodbridge as witnesses for Charlotte Howard Cullen. This document confirms that Charlotte likely had Dr. Bohannon's support. I could find no evidence whether a divorce took place prior to Dr. Cullen's death in 1849 so I presume it did not happen.

It is interesting that Charlotte wrote several letters to Simon Cullen, John's brother. She asked Simon to deliver them to John. Also a letter from John to Charlotte mentions he received her letter from his brother Simon. Up to now there was no evidence John even had a brother. So where did John's brother come from? What is he doing in Richmond? More crumbs to follow and mysteries to unravel. For now let's just consider John's domestic situation.

Marital difficulties often target people who have demanding careers. A host of potential pitfalls could have befallen John Cullen as he became exhausted after decades of accomplishments and demands. As a doctor he had access to many types of drugs and Charlotte did as well. Drugs were commonly stored at home for emergency situations. In the early 1800's laws did not regulate access to drugs. Often alcohol was used to escape stress, possibly over decades. We know today that such use not only affects kidney and liver functions but also causes significant brain damage. Mental damage can produce bizarre behavior that is considered abuse by today's standards.

The OSD evidence has partially answered questions about drug and alcohol use by the Cullen's. As mentioned on the previous pages as well as in the footnotes, this wonderful evidence, in the form of hand written letters by Charlotte Cullen as well as some written deposition questions by her lawyer, have provided a rare glimpse into the real workings of an 1840's doctor and his family. It is not a surprise that their problems are not much different than the problems families face today in the 21st century.

So, in summary these materials claim:

- *John Cullen had a serious alcohol drinking problem and had been advised to seek help from the "temperance society" by several of Charlotte's witnesses*

- *Charlotte Cullen admits to using opium for approximately 8 years (prior to 1844) to escape the results of John's drinking and the resulting personality changes and abuse*

- *John Cullen's drinking problem had noticeable health changing issues as early as 1838*

- *John Cullen became a mean spirited and nasty person when not drinking and failed to recognize his deteriorating mental and physical condition*

- *John Cullen physically assaulted Charlotte (by choking her after breaking down her bedroom door in a rage)*

- *John mentally abused Charlotte and several of his children over many years*

- *John Cullen believed his wife's health was unreasonable and his actions were justified (see John Cullen's handwritten letter of May 19th, 1846, Brock Collection, Huntingdon Library, San Marino, Ca. BR Box 33 (38))*

Remember, Dr. John Cullen has not presented any substantial viewpoint or defenses to his wife's claims. So this narrative is one sided from which we are trying to distill the truth, nearly 170 years later.

At least one side of the story exists. More often than not, both sides are missing and researchers are reduced to speculating. That is why it is so important for historians and researchers to label their work as one of many possible theories in such cases. Authority should not be claimed until significant evidence and proof is compiled, is cross checked, and any circumstantial claims have a factual basis, (OSD, etc.).

The OSD containing the Charlotte Cullen factual claims is located in the: *Brock Collection, Huntington Library, San Marino, Ca. – BR Box 33 (46) and one letter by John in BR Box 33 (38).*

Recall in the biography by Dr. Pollard, the cause of death of Dr. Cullen was thought to be "*softening of the brain,* hastened by being "*bled*". Based on this fragmentary description of the cause of death and a few other facts mentioned above, a number of possible theories about the death of Dr. John Cullen present themselves.

Dr. Cullen's death may have been due to natural causes - but could it also have been due to some unknown infection since he was routinely around sick patients? Or could it have been caused by a disease such as cancer or a brain tumor – that was untreatable at that time? Dr Pollard claimed he witnessed Dr Cullen using snuff tobacco on a regular basis before each of his lectures at the Medical College of Virginia as stated in his biography on page 194.

Or could it have been from a more salacious cause such as drugs or alcohol – or even a possible poisoning? Could it have been a murder in 1849? Is it possible John may have committed suicide? Although, it is less likely Dr. Cullen succumbed from any of the more sensational causes – they are possible given the evidence discovered so far.

From the OSD evidence, I believe the most likely cause of death was due to complications from heavy drinking for much of John Cullen's adult life. However, it is for you, the reader, to ponder and decide since the OSD facts are strong but not conclusive as of yet. We now have many new crumbs to follow in our trail to the tale, maybe even a historic CSI investigation?

Having formed a flesh and bones picture of John Cullen, let's turn our attention to other clues. The artifact that started all this awaits our attention.

5.2

Waiting 187 Years

The mere existence of this artifact (egg bottle), is a fabulous thread in and of itself - having tales that weave forward and backward as well. Following our thread and analyzing the likely scenarios of how it came to exist – leads us to a well known marketing genius of that era – Thomas W. Dyott. He built the largest industrial conglomerate in Philadelphia at that time – he was the Bill Gates of that era. His advertisements spanned the country and filled Philadelphia newspapers. John Cullen, in 1818, was located at "NE corner of 2nd & Chestnut Streets", only a few blocks from T.W. Dyott who was at the "NE corner of 2nd & Race Streets". He would surely have known him. Dyott was also a pharmacist and claimed to be a physician as well. However in his case, "MD" was likely added without credentials.

Why consider T.W.Dyott as being the most probable candidate related to our egg bottle (artifact)? Well, it is important not to dismiss an obvious answer – especially if it outweighs all other candidates to be considered. That is why we will investigate the strongest lead first, (most of the time). Over thousands of years, such an analysis paradigm has proved to work fastest. Let's not forget, we have many more tales to discover. Therefore time is important.

Thomas W. Dyott may be the answer we are looking for. Although "*original source documents*" confirm 99% of the facts needed to answer questions about the source of our artifact, there is an outside chance another possible theory could be correct. This is because the OSD do not specifically mention John Cullen and Thomas W. Dyott together. Such an "*original source document*" (OSD) would be 100% conclusive. We are very close as you can see by the evidence in the OSD mentioned below - perhaps further research may someday uncover such a document. So, recall the questions posed in a previous chapter (listed below).

- ***Where was the artifact made?***
- ***Who made the artifact? (What company?)***
- ***Are the artifact's characteristics (color, weight, lip style, etc.) similar to artifacts of known local origin? If so what glasshouses?***
- ***How long in time, was the artifact manufactured?***
- ***Is there evidence this style of bottle was made for others?***

Newspaper advertisements from 1816 through 1822 are the likely place to start since other researchers cite many OSD related to T.W. Dyott. Also, Philadelphia directories from 1818 through 1820 have large graphic ads by Dyott. Lastly books exist about Dyott and have OSD information in their "bibliography".

So, I'm off to the library again with high hopes and a happy heart. One does not need money to enjoy such a beautiful day. To park for free will require I enjoy a little bit more of this beautiful day than I had anticipated – about 15 blocks worth of enjoyment. Oh well, I'm finally at the front door and quickly sign in. The librarians seem to know just what I will be searching and have my 1817 and 1818 "*Aurora General Advertiser*" newspapers ready for me. Today I believe a segmented search pattern will be the best choice (I have no specific dates of interest – just very general ranges).

First I try April dates in 1818. From my previous searches in Philadelphia daily newspapers, I know "*Thomas W. Dyott*" had ads in most editions throughout the year. The ads vary from small to large, offering for sale, druggist items, household goods, hardware items, glassware and pottery, and food items. Some ads list his agents throughout the United States and North America. Others describe his relationship to various glasshouses. The size and scope of his business interests are impressive even today. Even so, it is not likely we will find our type of bottle listed, so our research is a long shot at best.

After searching 1818 and 1819 day by day, nothing of consequence is found. Discouraged, but not defeated, I try another newspaper covering the same period (1818 - 1819) - *"The Union, United States Gazette and True American, published by Bronson and Smith, 67 Dock St. corner Bank St."*

On April 4th, 1818, Dyott advertises he is sole agent for all the glassware of *Union, Olive, & Gloucester Glass Factories*, which can be seen at his store at the corner of Second & Race Streets. Dyott also lists many types of glassware he regularly carries. "Calcined Magnesia bottles" are listed in 1818 newspapers but not our type of bottle. The three listed glassworks are all located in southern New Jersey.

Let's move on to the next segment of my search. I've chosen, November 1819. On Saturday, November 13, 1819, Dyott advertises he is sole agent for *Olive, Gloucester and Kensington Glass Manufactories.* The list of glassware includes "*Liquid Magnesia Bottles*". The ad is run daily from October 28, 1819 through November 28, 1819.

My work has paid off again. I can hardly believe this wonderful direct evidence - perhaps John Cullen is no longer ordering bottles from Thomas Dyott. Maybe John Cullen has chosen to practice medicine rather than handle his Chemical and Druggist business (as the directory entries suggest)? Dyott appears to be reusing the mold by removing Cullen's name.

Liquid magnesia bottles were not just a sideline as illustrated by T. W. Dyott's 1820 Catalogue. They are listed as one of his regular glass items, available at all times. Under the category "*Flint and Other Glass Ware*", is listed "*Liquid Magnesia do*" bottles (between "*Seltzer Water do*" and "*Cologne Water do*"). The catalogue was published throughout April, May, and June of 1820. For example, on May 1, 1820 the Philadelphia newspaper, "*Aurora General Advertiser*" devotes nearly half a page to Dyott's catalogue.

Thomas W. Dyott continued advertising "*Liquid Magnesia Bottles*" on and off until around 1824 when it ceased and is not advertised again. Regardless, Dyott is selling egg bottles under the contents name, rather than by shape. This is likely the reason why so many researchers failed to discover the origins of the first marked mineral water bottle and the earliest known marked egg bottle. In fact, American egg bottles of this era have only been speculated about, never seen. This is the first, so far as I know.

Noted researchers "*Helen McKearin & Kenneth Wilson*" stated they believed egg bottles were not produced commercially in the United States before the 1840's. Many other researchers have reference quoted them over and over again, as if it was fact. We now know this theory to be incorrect. By way of illustration this can be seen in their book *American Bottles & Flasks and Their Ancestry* on page 240, as well as other books each has written individually.

It may be the United States, rather than Britain, was the origin of the first marked egg bottle, (*See Appendix C*). What about claims that "*William Hamilton*", obtained an early English patent for this type of bottle? Upon reading the actual English patents, "Hamilton" did not patent an egg bottle, but rather a process for filling them with mineral water. This can be seen in the original "*William Hamilton*" patent of 1809 No. 3232 titled "*A New Mode of Preparing Soda and other Mineral Waters, Spirituous, Acetous, Saccharine, Aromatic Liquers, and Sundry Improvements relative thereto*". Likewise Hamilton's patent of 1814, No. 3819, is titled "*Manufacture of Soda Water & c.*" with no mention about bottles in the text. Neither patent was for an "egg bottle" or any other type of container, or the mineral water itself.

So the egg bottle was never patented in England. There are so many references to similar bottles throughout history (pottery, metal, and glass) it would be hard to get a patent, simply because it would be considered "*known information*" and therefore not patentable. (*See Appendix C for other early patent examples as well.*)

There are claims egg glass bottles existed in the late 1700's in England. I find this unlikely because of the lack of archaeological confirmation in Europe. The rarest of black glass seal bottles are found archaeologically in England - from the1600's through 1820's – why not egg bottle artifacts (or pieces) - if they existed in this early period? The earliest historically documented commercial use of egg bottles in England dates around 1821. *(See: Schweppes earliest invoices offering glass bottles for sale - Appendix C).* One of these rare early egg bottles is embossed vertically, "*J. Schweppe & Co. / Genuine Superior / Aerated Waters / 79 Margaret St*". It is pontilled. All known examples have a narrow top ring or blob attached and flat base.

Thus the Cullen egg bottle is likely the oldest known marked mineral water bottle in the United States and possibly England as well.

Our oval shaped, egg bottle (opposite) is light bodied with a sheared top with neck ring. The ring is ¼' wide and the base is round with a circular open pontil. The top is characteristic of the 1700's when sheared lips and narrow glass neck rings were found more commonly on glass bottles. The glass color and density closely resemble other early period American marked glass from the Kensington transition period (after 1817 and before 1819).

The Dyott "*family medicine*" bottle pictured on the top of the next page was dug by myself in layer with archaeological context between 1815 and 1820, (*context of heavy lead glass Keene Sunburst Flask, and early mocha pottery - turned, buff bodied, cats eye, etc.*). It may be the earliest known "Dyott-Robertson family medicine bottle and would likely have preceded our egg bottle by a few years since it has no tool markings on the neck below the lip area and characteristics are more common to the period before 1817. Tool marks are obvious on all other known examples of the Dyott-Robertson bottles. Tool markings generally were a later process (1818–1838) which corresponded to when Dyott owned the Kensington glassworks. The neck of the early variant is only 5/8 of an inch, quite short when compared to other known examples - the glass is much lighter in weight and appears to be of much higher quality as well. Less dense and higher quality glass generally distinguishes glass artifacts from early southern New Jersey glasshouses as opposed to those produced by Dyott's Kensington. The picture at the bottom of the next page contains the earliest known marked T.W. Dyott bottle between two Dyott-Robertson bottles of different eras. It is made of white glass (not lead glass – but often mistakenly called flint glass) with an archaeological and historical context between 1809 and 1815. This is the only known clear (white) glass T.W. Dyott medicine bottle known to me. Perhaps there are others, but at this time unknown to myself and other researchers.

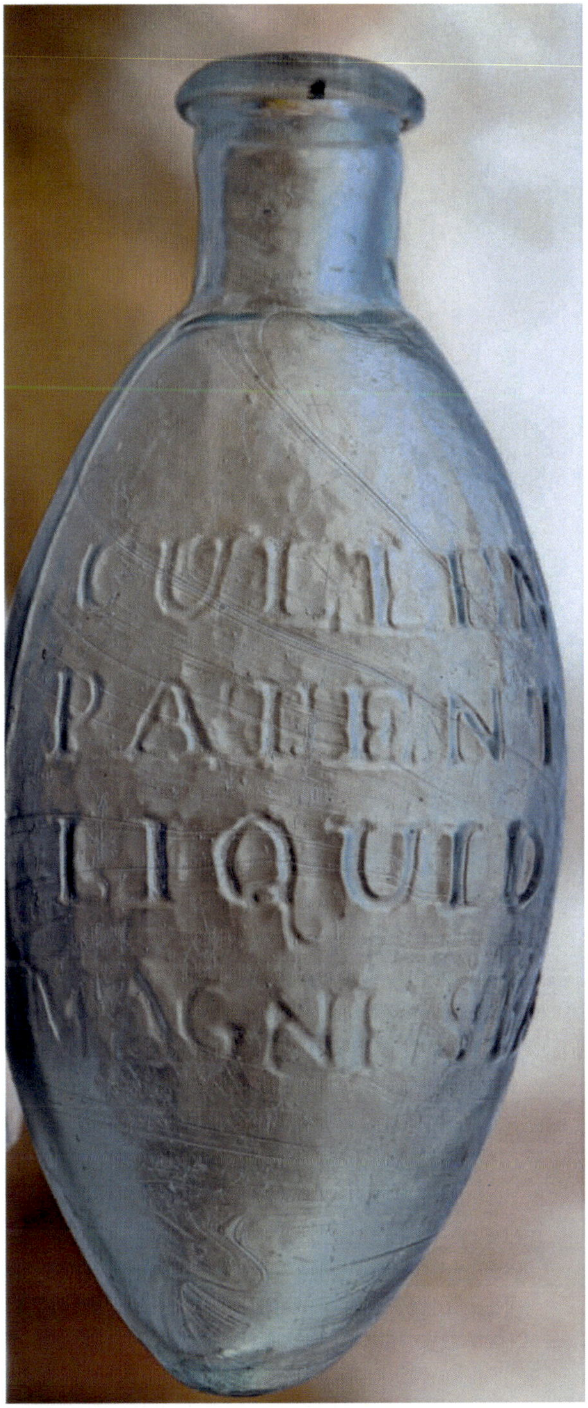

"Cullen's Patent Liquid Magnesia"

Approximately 2-11/16 inch body width, 6-1/8 inch high, ¼ inch string neck ring, round base with open pontil, sheared neck 1/32 inch above string neck ring, color is distorted from its natural light green.

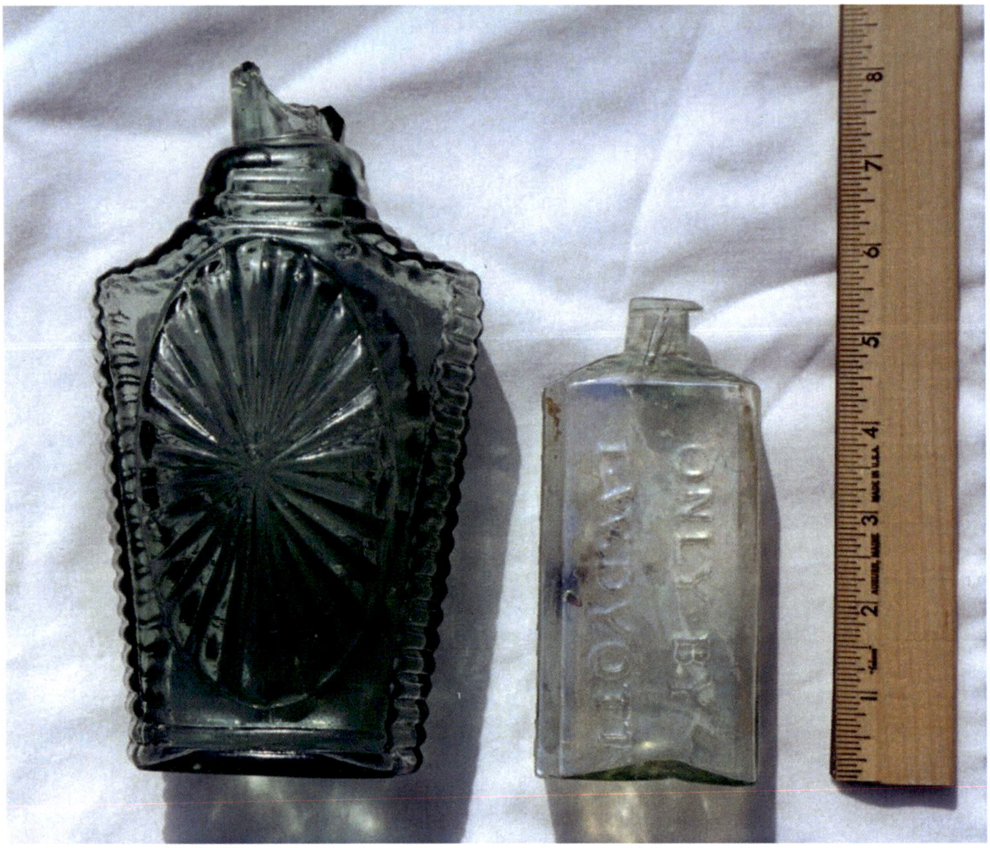

In center is: "*Dr. Robertson's Family medicines Sold Only by T.W. Dyott*"
Early "mushroom" style flared lip with no tool markings on the neck below the lip area.
Keene sunburst flask found in layer with "*Dyott*" - Archaeological context is between 1815 and 1820.

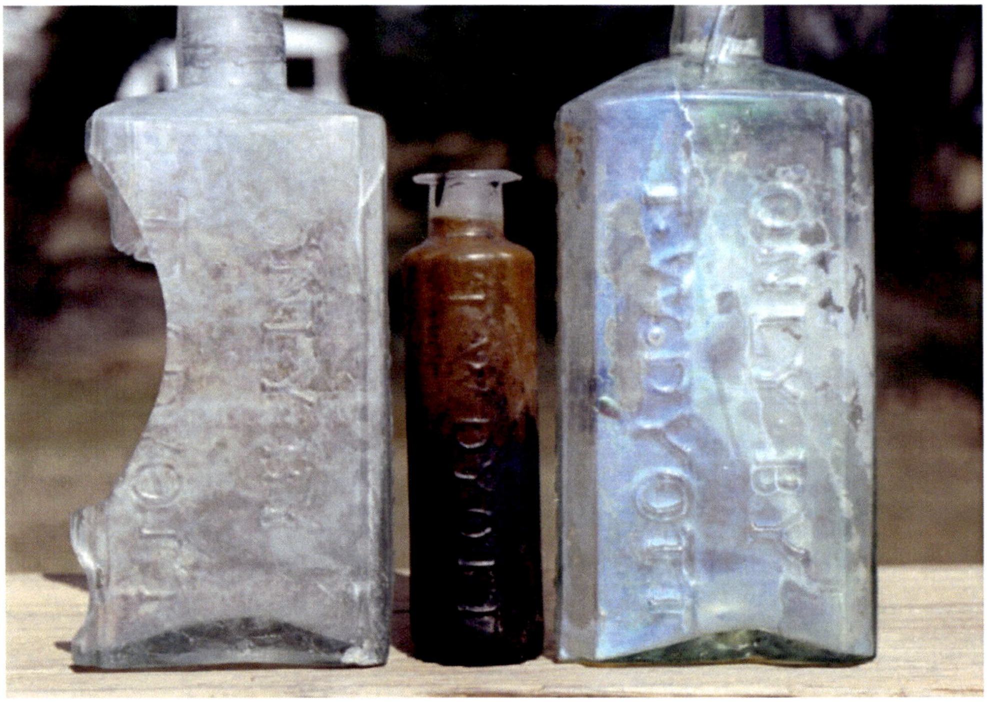

In center is a white glass bottle marked *T.W.Dyott,* with archaeological context 1809 – 1815.

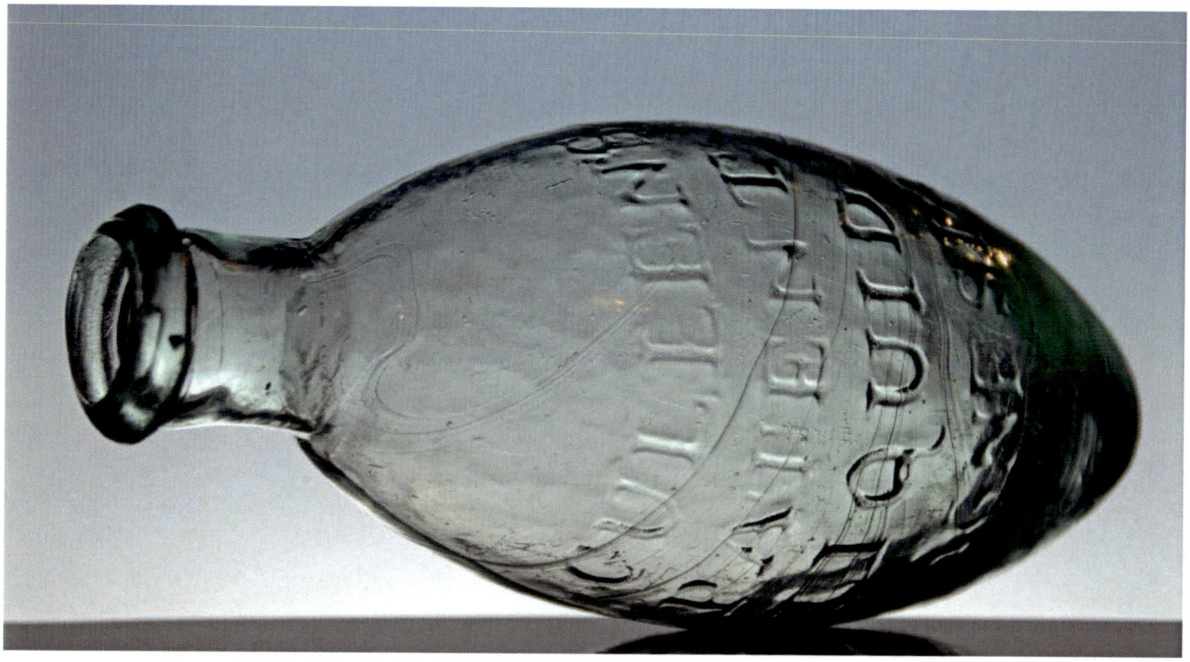

Another view of the *"Cullen's Patent Liquid Magnesia"* – Note: sheared lip protruding above the neck ring.

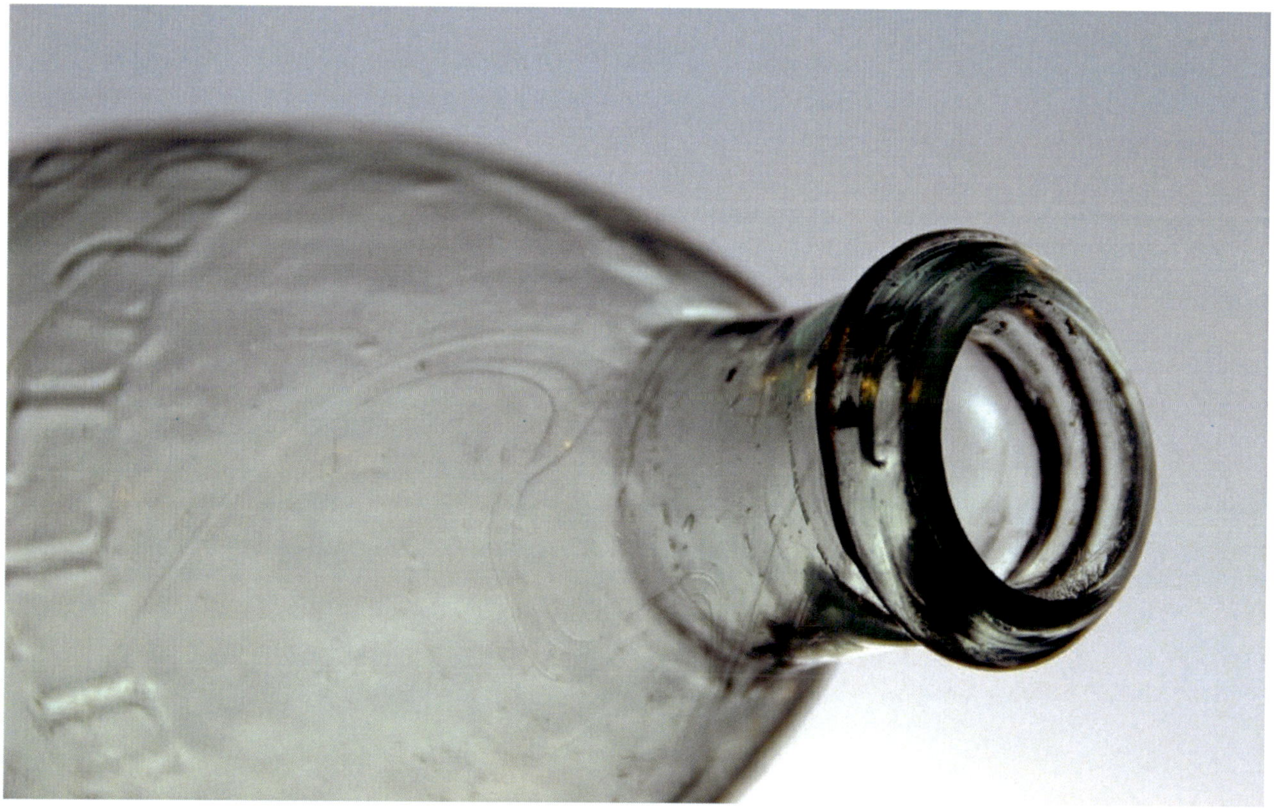

Close up view of the lip and neck of Cullen's egg bottle – color is accurate in these photographs

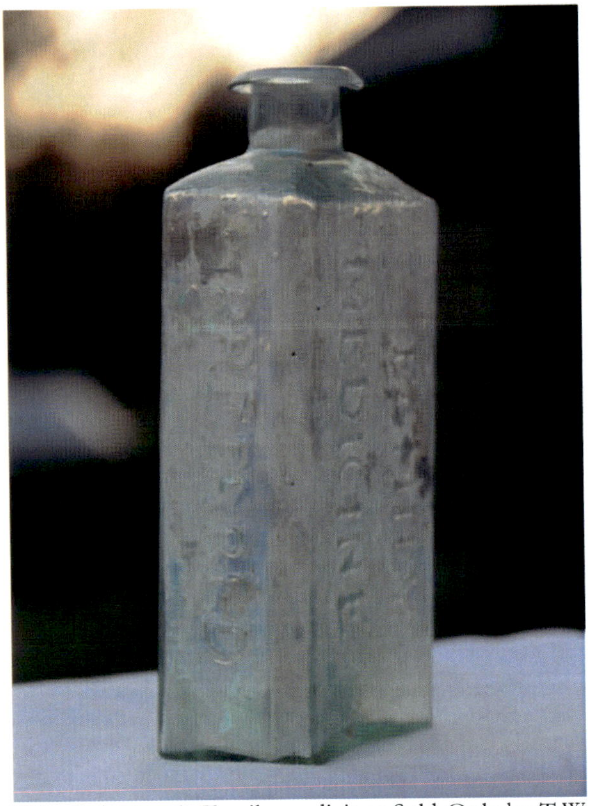

"Dr. Robertson's Family medicines Sold Only by T.W. Dyott" - Likely made in one of agent Dyott's south Jersey glass factories - Archaeological context 1815 – 1820, Context by characteristics, design, and properties 1810 - 1815.

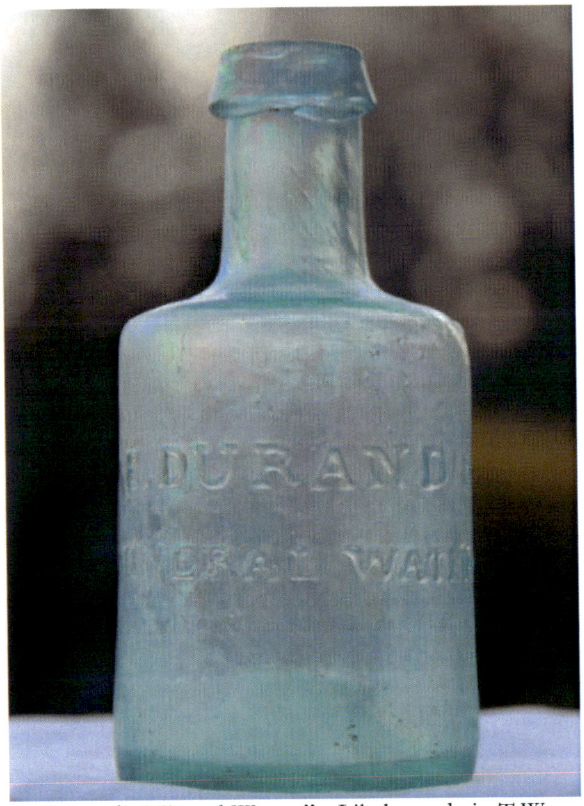

"E Durand's Mineral Waters" - Likely made in T.W. Dyott's Kensington, Philadelphia glass factory while under his ownership - Archaeological context 1827 – 1833, Historical context 1825 – 1833. (Height 5 ¼ in. width 2 9/16 in., other examples not pictured, vary in height from 5 1/8 to 5 5/16 in.).

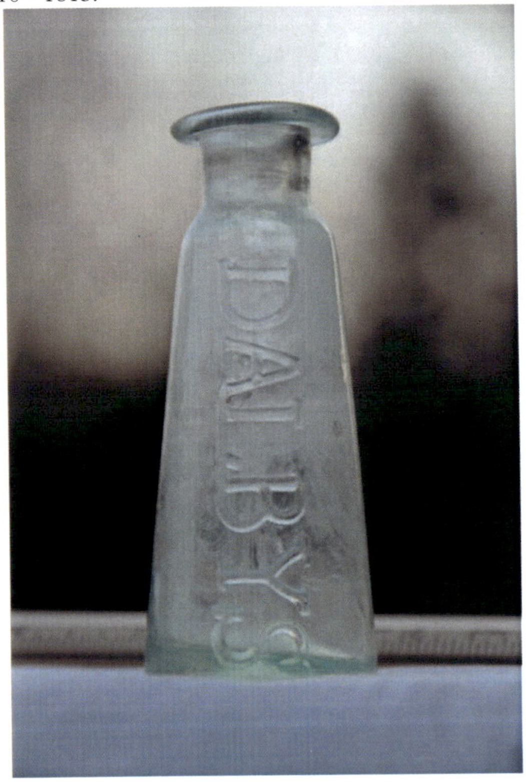

"Dalby's Carminitive" – Likely made in south Jersey or early Philadelphia glass manufactory - Archaeological context 1790 – 1805 (prior to Dyott), Context by characteristics, design, and properties 1790 – 1810. Embossed lettering tapers top to bottom, mixed orientation, large size, and inward double folded lip. (Height 4 in. base diameter 1 9/16 in.)

All artifacts pictured have a complete provenience and are shown prior to any preservation. All were recovered in Philadelphia, in layer, by your author.

All marked English torpedo or egg bottles date from 1821 through 1890, (*Appendix C*). This is equally true of US marked mineral water bottles. In fact, the only known 1820's marked US mineral water bottles (*E. Durand's Mineral Waters* – a cylinder type bottle in two different mold styles) could not have been produced before 1825 because Elias Durand did not move to Philadelphia from Baltimore until at least 1825. My digging experience on three occasions is that the associative archaeological context of "*E. Durand*" bottles is always 1827 through 1833 - much later than our "*Dr. Cullen*" egg bottle artifact.

If Schweppes egg bottles are not found archaeologically in England before the early 1820's - Why? This is largely because Schweppes owners built a mineral water manufacturing facility in Derby (at Friar Gate) in 1812. It was next to the stoneware potters of Derbyshire who supplied the pottery mineral water bottles they used. The stoneware bottles could be manufactured by the potters then filled immediately with mineral water - eliminating the shipping cost and danger of explosions. This would enable Schweppes to sell their mineral water cheaper than competitors and run a smoother manufacturing operation because there would be less chance of disruption due to accidents. Such a production cost advantage would have been lost if glass bottling commenced before they gained market dominance and the danger of explosion eliminated. So they continued for some time using stoneware bottles.

Two other English mineral water makers, Nicholas Paul and William Hamilton also used earthenware bottles in the pre-1825 period. Archaeological evidence in the form of a marked pottery bottle (without the EX tax code) exists for Nicholas Paul. Hamilton claims to have used both pottery and glass containers in a description of his manufacturing process in 1809, but no archaeological evidence of glass has been found.

Why did the switchover to glass bottles eventually occur?

1.) First, the stoneware bottles were too porous limiting the shelf life of the product, (it became flat);

2). Second, Schweppe & Co. became the official supplier of mineral water to the entire royal family after 1835. Thus, they acquired market dominance. A royal endorsement is hard to overcome. They could now improve the product's quality and absorb the increased cost of the glass bottles. The earliest marked Schweppe & Co. glass egg bottle has the "*79 Margaret St*" address embossed on it and Schweppes invoices from 1821 are the first to mention these bottles;

3). The third and most important reason for the switchover is that the technology needed to load light weight glass egg bottles became available. A much more precise remote controlled type of liquid pressure safety valve had been invented in the US in 1817 such that mineral water apparatus could fill glass bottles without danger of explosion – previously, pottery bottles were used because they were far stronger and could absorb a far wider range of pressures and mishandling. Such a valve was not patented until 1817 in the United States by James S. Ewing of Philadelphia. It took a few more years for the technology to travel overseas such that

"*Schweppe & Co.*" could experiment with it and ultimately copy it.

The switchover from pottery bottles began slowly around 1821 to 1830 in an attempt to increase the quality of the product. London directory entries show 79 Margaret St was used from 1809 through 1831. During these early years only limited bottling was tried due to technology limitations (the bottles and equipment had a tendency to explode). With new technology from the US (James S. Ewing) and with the Royal family choosing Schweppes as the official supplier of mineral waters in 1836, success grew quickly and costs were controlled - the switchover accelerated and pottery bottles were phased out. Most Schweppe egg bottles have the 51 Bernes & Oxford St. addresses, used from 1832 through 1895 and are not pontilled.

The magnitude of this switchover can be seen by considering the 1851 London World's fair. Schweppes & Co. sold over one million torpedo bottles of mineral water at the fair.

Even into the 20th century, grocery store clerks can relate many stories of glass soda bottles exploding on store shelves for no apparent reason. It wasn't until plastic bottles came into widespread use in the 1980's that the problem largely disappeared from American grocery stores.

Clearly if modern technology, 150 years later, failed to eliminate the problem, it must have been nearly impossible for the pioneers of the early soda water industry to resolve the situation.

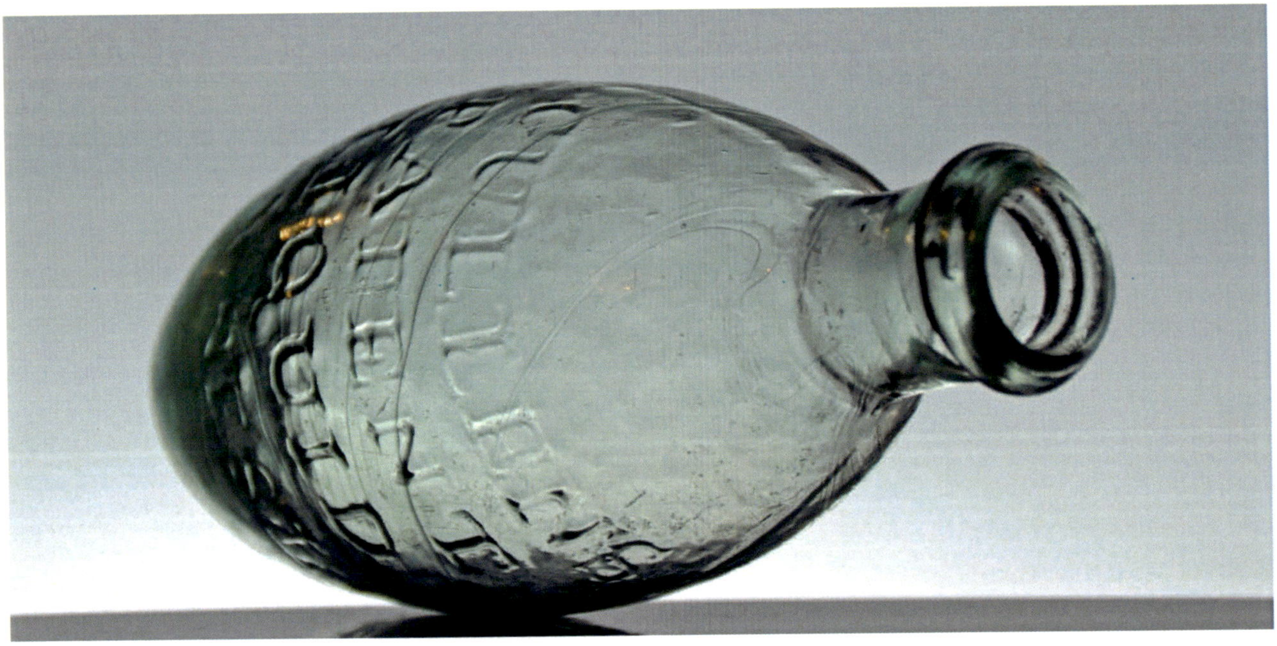

The first American embossed, light weight, artificial mineral water bottle – likely made in Dyott's Kensington glass factory, Philadelphia Pa. – approximately April – November, 1818.

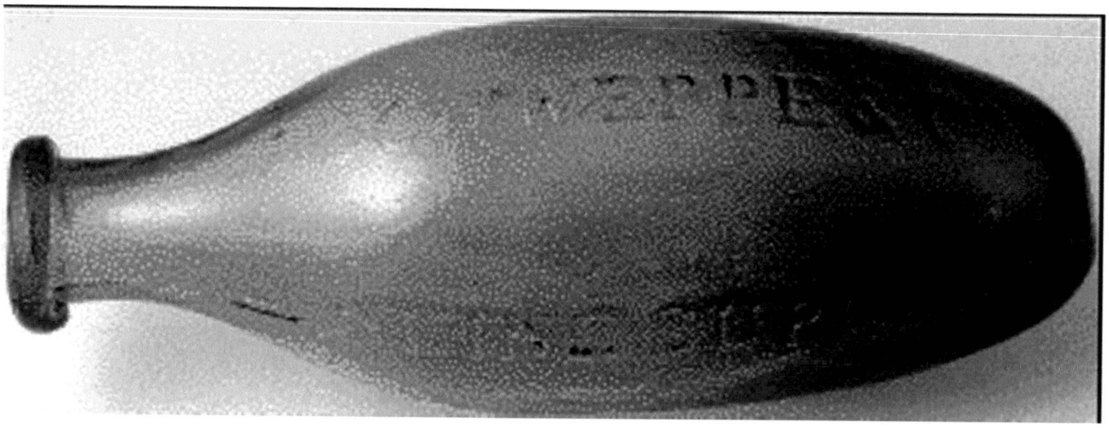

"J. Schweppe & Co. / Genuine Superior / Aerated Waters / 79 Margaret St".
Schweppes earliest known marked bottle and earliest marked English egg bottle circ. approximately 1821 – 1831

According to the "*Post Office London Directories by B. Critchett*" and others, "*79 Margaret St.*" was used by *Schweppe & Co.* from approximately 1809 to 1831. Then Schweppe & Co moved to 51 Bernes & Oxford Streets from 1832 until 1895. Before 1809, Schweppe's addresses were 75 Margaret St. (1798-1808), 11 Margaret St. (1795-1798), 8 Kings St., Holborn (1795), and 141 Drury Lane (1792-1794).

However, the earliest known Schweppes invoices, offering glass egg bottles for sale, in addition to their normal stoneware bottles, are dated 1821, *(See Appendix C)*. The dark color, flatted base, density, weight, and sand pontil are all consistent with many other known examples from the 1820's and 1830's in both England and the United States, *(See Rushton & Aspinwall / No 86 William St / & 110 Broadway / New York, circ 1833 – 1837)*

During this early period of use (1821-1825), bottling in glass egg bottles was likely more experimental and then slowly grew in popularity because of the improved shelf life of the mineral water as compared to Schweppes normal stoneware bottled mineral waters. As manufacturing improvements began to prevent explosions, commercial level glass bottling became practical in the mid 1820's. Schweppes and others in the early 1820's began offering glass bottled mineral water, even though it cost more, as an alternative to their traditional stoneware bottles. The public supported the new glass egg bottle since the product was preserved better and the company had far less returns for bad or lost product - so it was a win / win situation for everyone – customer and company.

Prevention of explosions was what allowed the glass egg bottle to be used, not the repeal of two English taxes as historians have long believed (*English glass tax (1745-1845); English medicine (soda water) tax (1804-1833)*). Clearly the taxes had not been repealed in the 1820's when commercial level glass egg bottling began.

June 9—dtf

THE SUBSCRIBER,

Being appointed Sole Agent for the Union, Olive and Gloucester

Glass Factories,

HAS constantly on hand, a large and general assortment of first and second quality WINDOW GLASS, of the following different sizes : 6 by 8—7 by 9—8 by 10—9 by 11—9 12—10 by 12—12 by 16—14 by 18— 16 by 20—18 by 22—30 by 24, &c.

ALSO,

Vials from half ounce to eight ounces, Essence Peppermint, Bateman's Stroughton's Godfrey's, British Oil, Turlington's, Dalby's Balsam of Honey, Duffey's Haerlem Oil, Opodeldock and Essence Vials, Mustard, Cayenne Pepper, and Snuff Bottles, Seltzer, Cologne Water and Pocket Bottles, Confectioner's Preserving Bottles, Show Glasses, &c.

The first quality Glass, from either of the above factories, is equal to any made in the U. States, and will at all times be sold in quantities at the lowest manufacturer's prices.

T. W. Dyott, *Druggist,*

Corner of Second & Race streets, Philadelphia.

Who has on hand, in addition to the above, a large and complete assortment of fresh Drugs, Medicines, Patent Medicines, Paints, Dye Stuffs, &c. &c. any of which he will supply country merchants, druggists and manufacturers, at very reduced prices, for cash or on the usual credit, or in barter for any of the following articles of produce:—Flour, flaxseed, oil, rye and apple whiskey, rye and buckwheat meal, pork, beef, fish, butter, cheese, lard, beeswax, pearl and pot ashes, rum, sugar, rice, cotton, &c.

NB. Window Glass of any size, and hollow ware of every description, made to order at a few days' notice.

Dec 25 dtf

It cannot be made too

Olive, Gloucester, & Kensington Glass Manufactories,

(IN BLAST.)

THE Subscribers respectfully inform their friends and their customers, that they have now commenced new Blasts at the above manufactories, and will be happy to receive orders for any of the following description of Hollow Glass Ware and Window Glass; for the sale of which, and for receiving all orders, they have appointed Dr. T. W. DYOTT, Druggist, their *sole agent*, with whom all the Glass as it is manufactured, will be deposited for sale, by which means, from the extensive stock generally on hand, almost every order can be executed at an hour's notice.

The following is a list of the articles generally on hand, viz:—

Gallon bottles	Essence vials
Half gallons, quarts	Durable inks
Pint pockets	Balsam of honey
Half pint do	Jesuits
Gallon round N. Mo.	Daffy's
Half gallon do.	Harlem oil
Pints, half pints	Cephalic snuffs
Gallon round W. Mo.	Bateman's
Half gallons, quarts	British oils
Pints, half pints	Peppermints
Gallon jars turned	Stoughton's
Half gallons	Godfrey's
Quarts, pints	Dalby's
Gallon jars straight	Turlington's
Half gallons	Opodeldocs
Quarts, pints	Salt Mou. ground stopper bottles from 4 oz. to 2 gallons
Claret bottles	Tincture bottles, grd. stoppers, from 1 oz. to 2 gallons
Sweet oil do.	Specie bottles with tin covers, from 4 oz. to 3 gallons
Seltzer water do.	Show globes
Liquid Magnes do.	Funnels
Olive do.	Mortars and pestals
Caper do.	Breast pipes
Anchovie do.	Nipple shells
Brandy fruits	Nursing bottles
Maccabou snuff do.	Cupping glasses
Rappee do.	Urinals
Scotch do. lb & ½ lb	Smelling bottles
Blacking bottles	Lamp glasses
Mustard do.	Clock do.
do. do. London	Window glass, all sizes
Kians	
Essence mustard botls.	
Cologne water do.	
Camphor matrasses	
Retorts	
Vials from ½ to 8 oz.	

DAVID WOLF & Co.
Olive Glass Works.
JONA. HAINES,
Gloucester Glass Works.
HEWSON & CONNELL,
Kensington Glass Works.

T W Dyott. *Sole Agent,*

North East corner of Second & Race streets, Philadelphia.

Who has for sale or barter, at very reduced prices, a general assortment of Drugs, Medicines, Dye Stuffs, Colours, &c. suitable for supplying country merchants, druggists, physicians, and manufacturers.

Oct. 28—dtf.

Dr. Vickers's Ointment for the Tetter, etc.

Thomas W. Dyott's ads from 1819

The 1st newspaper image appeared July 1, 1819 in the, "*The Union, United States Gazette and True American*" of Philadelphia, Pennsylvania and mentions Dyott is agent for Union, Olive, and Gloucester glassworks. No mention of Liquid Magnesia bottles between Seltzer & Cologne bottles. The 2nd newspaper image in the same newspaper appeared November 14, 1819 (page 4, col. 3) and now lists Liquid Magnesia bottles under Seltzer bottles. Dyott is now agent for Olive, Gloucester, and Kensington glassworks.

Courtesy of "*The Library Company of Philadelphia*"

(Call number 4-B-1 [567.F])

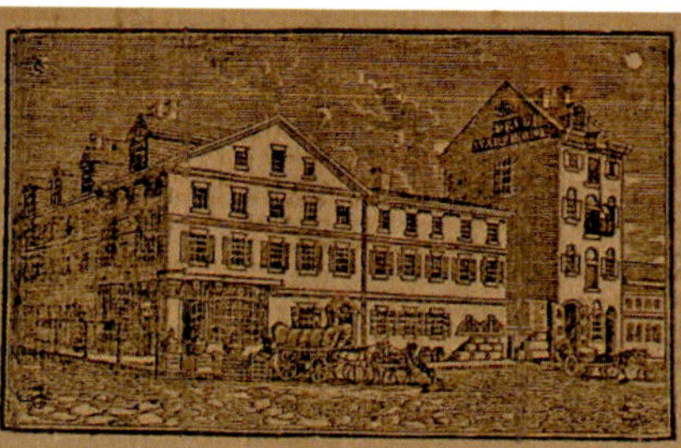

CATALOGUE

OF DRUGS & MEDICINES, PATENT MEDICINES, DYE STUFFS, COLORS, GLASS WARE, AND SUNDRY ARTICLES,

FOR SALE OR BARTER BY DR. T. W. DYOTT,

AT THE PHILADELPHIA DRUG & FAMILY MEDICINE WAREHOUSE, N. E. CORNER OF SECOND AND RACE STS.

DRUGS, &c.

PATENT MEDICINES, &c.

SUNDRIES.

FLINT AND OTHER GLASS WARE.

DYE STUFFS, COLORS, &c.

JAMES BEDFORD, New Orleans, General Agent for T. W. DYOTT.

Thomas W. Dyott's Catalog 1820

This newspaper image appeared May 1, 1820 in the, "*Aurora General Advertiser*" of Philadelphia, Pennsylvania (page 4). It shows a woodcut graphic of Dyott's buildings in Philadelphia as well as the regular items he sells. It mentions "*Liquid Magnesia*" bottles are part of his regular inventory of bottles for sale.

(See next page for blowup of the section where these bottles are mentioned, titled "*Flint and other Glassware*".)

Courtesy of "*The Library Company of Philadelphia*"

(Call number 4-B-3-5)

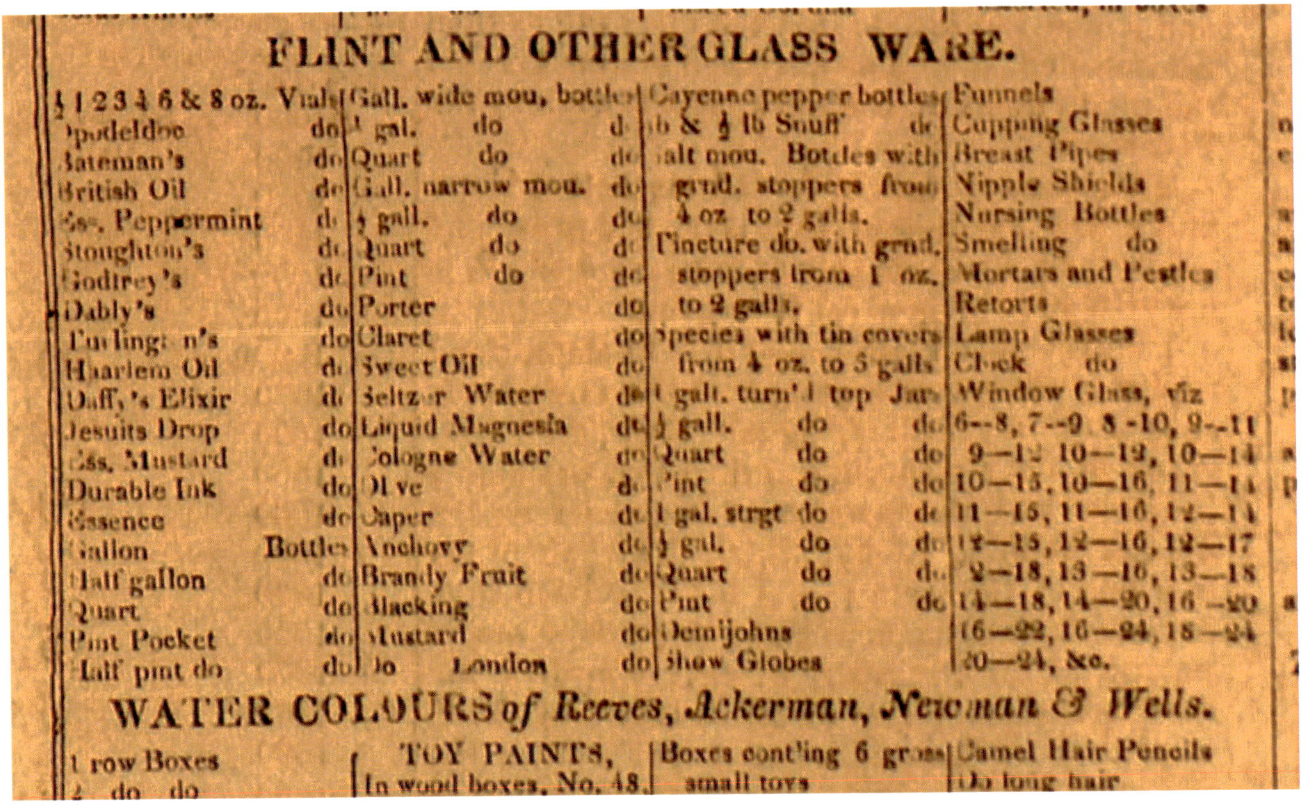

FLINT AND OTHER GLASS WARE.

½ 1 2 3 4 6 & 8 oz. Vials	Gall. wide mou. bottles	Cayenne pepper bottles	Funnels
Opodeldoc do	½ gal. do do	lb & ½ lb Snuff do	Cupping Glasses
Bateman's do	Quart do do	Salt mou. Bottles with	Breast Pipes
British Oil do	Gall. narrow mou. do	grnd. stoppers from	Nipple Shields
Ess. Peppermint do	½ gall. do do	4 oz to 2 galls.	Nursing Bottles
Stoughton's do	Quart do do	Tincture do. with grnd.	Smelling do
Godfrey's do	Pint do do	stoppers from 1 oz.	Mortars and Pestles
Dably's do	Porter do	to 2 galls.	Retorts
Turlington's do	Claret do	Species with tin covers	Lamp Glasses
Haarlem Oil do	Sweet Oil do	from 4 oz. to 5 galls	Clock do
Daffy's Elixir do	Seltzer Water do	1 gall. turn'd top Jars	Window Glass, viz
Jesuits Drop do	Liquid Magnesia do	½ gall. do do	6--8, 7--9 8-10, 9--11
Ess. Mustard do	Cologne Water do	Quart do do	9—12 10—12, 10—14
Durable Ink do	Olive do	Pint do do	10—15, 10—16, 11—14
Essence do	Caper do	1 gal. strgt do do	11—15, 11—16, 12—14
Gallon Bottles	Anchovy do	½ gal. do do	12—15, 12—16, 12—17
Half gallon do	Brandy Fruit do	Quart do do	12—18, 13—16, 13—18
Quart do	Blacking do	Pint do do	14—18, 14—20, 16—20
Pint Pocket do	Mustard do	Demijohns	16—22, 16—24, 18—24
Half pint do do	Do London do	Show Globes	20—24, &c.

WATER COLOURS *of Reeves, Ackerman, Newman & Wells.*

1 row Boxes	TOY PAINTS,	Boxes cont'ing 6 gross	Camel Hair Pencils
2 do do	In wood boxes, No. 48.	small toys	Do long hair

From Thomas W. Dyott's cataloge of 1820

This newspaper image appeared May 1, 1820 in the, "*Aurora General Advertiser*" of Philadelphia, Pennsylvania (page 4) and was part of the larger catalogue of all items that was printed on most of the page. It mentions "Liquid Magnesia" bottles are part of his regular inventory of bottles for sale (between Seltzer Water & Cologne Water bottles).

Courtesy of "*The Library Company of Philadelphia*"
(Call number 4-B-3-5)

5.3

A Historical Home Run

What questions remain open from our trail of clues (crumbs)? It is important not to quit our research too soon – determination and persistence pay off in the end. Often the most meaningful results are the last to be found. These later results tend to be of the smoking gun variety – even the strongest critic cannot overcome them. More often than not such records do not exist - but when the treasure is found, the excitement is overwhelming. The rarity of these situations is what drives historical researchers. These questions seem to remain.

- ***Are there other possible historical records in Philadelphia from Cullen's time period (1816 – 1822) besides directory entries? Such as: Newspapers, magazines, letters, journals, etc?***
- ***Was his Patented "Liquid Magnesia" the only mineral water he made?***
- ***Did he advertise his patented mineral water?***
- ***Was the mineral water sold in a soda fountain as well as bottles?***
- ***Did he have other sizes of bottles?***
- ***How much did he charge for the mineral water?***

Over the previous year, since finding our primary artifact I have tried and failed to locate any direct Philadelphia historical records related to it. Numerous visits to libraries and historical institutions had turned up nothing. The lone exception was the "patent" index records, found using other resources. Such a correlation would ordinarily be strong enough to reach conclusions of truth. My "error analysis" (scientific) instincts were fundamental however – the picture seemed incomplete. When the result is visible but how it came to be is not – review again and again your research. Go over and over it until you are comfortable with your work.

The early newspapers of Philadelphia in 1817 – 1819 seemed to hold the best hope. Searching early newspapers is overwhelming at first and one has a tendency to request too many volumes to sift through in a day. It is better to slow down and focus on less and you will generate better results. So over the year I continued searching persistently page by page.

I used segmented searches, targeted date searches, and binary searches. Searching the 1818 "Aurora General Advertiser" (a daily paper), I was using targeted date searches in April 1818, going forward day by day. The reason I targeted April through May 1818 is because our "patent" date is May 4, 1818.

Most issues contained 4 pages. After a while, a pattern emerges as to how the editor arranged items in his paper. Theatre items were in the top left area of the third page, legal notices and real estate were usually on page two, and page four usually contained the ads with graphics. Ads without graphics are found on all pages. Understanding this pattern helps to target your search efforts. Normally, I scan for more than just my current area of interest. This case was no exception, significant material involving other artifacts was found with wonderful tales of their own – but that is for other books.

In this early period of US history, the majority of businesses did not advertise because their market was limited to the local neighborhood where they were located. Any chance of hitting a historical home run (direct evidence of our artifact) is exceedingly small. However, the historical record discloses a very special person – John Cullen the visionary. So we must adjust our thinking in such cases - the normal case may not be true. Recall in an earlier chapter where I stated the following:

> "One must always adjust, should later evidence suggest a different answer to a question. Good error analysis will uncover the truth. So don't worry at this stage if you are later corrected by your research."

Our research has now corrected our thinking. Our newspaper search is far more worthwhile than normal. We are compelled to continue.

April seems unlikely since John Cullen had not yet received his patent. Regardless, we must check dates before his patent was issued on the outside chance that his business was already functional. Meaning Cullen's business was an "*end to end viable business*" - a working manufacturing process and a viable business product being sold retail or wholesale.

This does not seem possible given that his "*Chymical & Druggist*" business on "*NE corner of Chestnut & Second Street*" is listed for only two years, the year of his "*patent*" and the next, 1819. So, April is slowly checked day by day – still nothing and I am approaching the last day - I'm searching April, 29th 1818. Maybe I should move on and search June or July 1818, since early period communication was likely slow and this was not a matter of interest to a wide audience.

> However, I decide not to skip forward – I will continue to move forward through April and May methodically no matter what my preconceived ideas are! (Recall, from a previous chapter, this is the key skill needed for field work in archaeology, "*analysis skill*".)

The next day is April 30th, 1818. Page one has nothing, page two nothing, page three nothing, no wait a minute – what is this – "*Cullen's Liquid Magnesia*" in bold print and a long column printed under it. Forget page four for a moment – this is wonderful! I am bent over looking at the newspaper and the extraordinary rarity of this situation sweeps over me. Some researchers spend a lifetime and are not fortunate enough to discover a significant historical first. Given the early date, 1818, and the correlation to the artifact's raised lettering, without a doubt, this discovery has tremendous historical significance going forward from this moment in time.

The advertisement continued from day to day through May 19th, 1818, but was updated on May 7th, 1818 with the "*patent*" information, (granted May 4th, 1818), three days after it was granted. The speed the patent information traveled and was typeset (by hand) in an existing advertisement is surprising even by today's standards.

Without such a strong correlation with the newspapers of 1818, the significance of my artifact could easily have been overlooked and mischaracterized. Illustrating that, conclusions based on "second hand knowledge quoted from recent references" and not on "Original Source Documents (OSD)" is risky business. Without OSD many of the core questions raised by my artifact would be open to argument and some experts would impose their own fictional conclusions on the public, without knowing the archaeological context information. These mistaken conclusions would then be perpetuated by "*reference quoting*" so frequently, as to become truth to the unsuspecting public. The problem has become much worse because of the internet, where mistakes can be repeated exponentially. It is my experience, in this narrow field of concentration, when actually checking supposed facts supporting conclusions reached, the so called "facts" are often completely wrong.

Thus, it is extremely important to always check the original source documents (OSD) and not just accept some other person's statements, no matter how important their reputation. I expect no less from anyone referencing my work – and if found to be mistaken in any material fact – to be corrected. Know that I will celebrate your discovery and be happy for your good work. I will thank you for bringing me further illumination.

Lastly, it is important to leave the door open whenever your "*direct evidence search*" does not bear fruit. Clearly label your conclusions as one of many possible theories and let the reader determine if he sees another theory as more probable. Do not label yours as authoritative unless the OSD supports it in all significant material facts. Allow your peers to decide the relative strength of your arguments and theories when OSD support is minimal or non-existent.

Fortunately my OSD searches were highly successful, so in this case, I offer the following information as authoritative, referenced solely by OSD in all material facts. My conclusions likewise are authoritative since they are highly probable given the level of OSD corroboration herein. By way of illustration, the following is quoted from John Cullen's ad that follows herein. It shows the spectacular correlation with the artifact itself, describing the egg bottle exactly as it appears today including the embossed text in the glass. Further, it shows that multiple egg bottle sizes were available. A fact that was completely unknown until found here.

"…..The solution may be either drank at the fount (as mineral waters) at 12 ½ cents per half pint, or may be had in bottles of an oval shape of different sizes, marked in raised letters "Cullen's Liquid Magnesia", and labelled Cullen's Solution of Magnesia.
Observe none is genuine except what answers the above description, and is signed by the sole proprietor, **John Cullen**.
Price – large bottle $3 per doz. – small $2.
75 cents for the large, 50 for the small bottles, will be refunded on returning the empty bottles……."

This excerpt illustrates why early period glass artifacts are rarely found archaeologically in the US. A refund of 25% of the purchase price for the return of empty Cullen egg bottles is promised. Most were likely returned which tends to explain why so few early period glass artifacts were discarded.

For instance, the evidence from T.W. Dyott's glass house manifests and production inventories (*1815 thru 1820*) clearly show production of hundreds of thousands of bottles from the early US period. This is in stark contrast to what is actually found archaeologically - large quantities of pottery but very little glass.

This ratio of pottery to glass changes in the late 1820's and larger and larger quantities of glass are found while the proportion of pottery from year to year tends to stay the same. Clearly the glass became more of a throw away commodity as smaller and smaller money sums were offered for their return.

This question has troubled most early period researchers (both professional & amateur) and now has at least one plausible answer.

So let's move ahead to the specifics of John Cullen's advertisements, fully set forth in the following pages after a short introduction, followed by pictures of his ads from the Philadelphia newspaper, "*Aurora General Advertiser*" in 1818.

The most compelling and important historical context related to any artifact is always direct reference but so rarely encountered in this early period as to be exceptionally exciting when found.

Seldom is a historical home run hit. We have one here. Our artifact, John Cullen's Liquid Magnesia bottle, is specifically mentioned in John Cullen's newspaper advertisements of April 30, 1818 through May 19, 1818 in the Philadelphia "Aurora (Published Daily for William Duane 110 & 112 Walnut St. Phila.)". An extensive advertisement describes his invention (liquid magnesia) and why it is so different from other types of magnesia, who should use it, why it should be used, how to use it, culminating with a description of its availability (at his mineral water fountain and by large or small oval bottles with raised lettering, as well as pricing info, etc.). Note the egg (oval) bottle came in two sizes. On May 7, 1818 Cullen updated the first advertisement (of April 30 1818) with spelling corrections, paragraph indentation, and paragraph separation, as well as the addition of a new top line "*By Letters Patent From U. States*". It should be noted, many academic experts of early period US history suggest information traveled much more slowly. This scenario was likely true when extremely rural locations were involved. However, for Cullen's US patent of May 4 1818 to already be mentioned in a Philadelphia newspaper, far from Washington D.C. 3 days later on May 7, 1818, may be cause to rethink the spread of knowledge from region to region in this early US period.

On the next page is text of John Cullen's first and second advertisements from the Philadelphia newspaper "*Aurora General Advertiser*" published daily for William Duane 110 & 112 Walnut St.

First ad – April 30, 1818 through May 6, 1818
(no mention of his pending Patent)
Second ad – May 7, 1818 through May 19, 1818
(similar to the First ad with a few corrections)
(1st mention of his Patent – (granted May 4, 1818))
Third ad – May 20, 1818 through May 26, 1818
(also, mentions his Patent)

Generally all advertisements appeared on page three (of four total pages).

****

Ad numbers 1 & 2: ***(In the 2nd ad only slight spelling corrections, paragraph separation, and the patent line added at the top, as shown on the next page)***

By Letters Patent From the U. States

Cullen's Liquid Magnesia,

Approved and recommended by several of the most eminent Physicians of Philadelphia

The transparent solution of Magnesia is presented to the public with the sanction and particular recommendation of many of the most respectable Physicians of the city, as the most eligible mode of exhibiting Magnesia. The solution possesses the virtues of that medicine in an eminent degree – acts more speedily – with greater certainty and is not liable to form concretions in bowels, as messrs. Brande & Monroe have discovered, are sometimes produced by solid Magnesia. It combines with its antacid and aperient principles, the very desirable property of composing the stomach – allaying the excessive vomiting and carrying away the bile and offensive matter. Hence may be inferred its greater efficacy in the summer complaints of children, females, & c. To persons of bilious habits it is recommended as an excellent correction of bile and acidity – communicates tone to the stomach – operates as a gentle laxative and establishes a permanent and regular state of the bowels. A discretionary use of this agreeable beverage enables persons of every age, sex, and constitution, to keep their bowels moderate without the use of salts or drastic purges (hitherto used) which never fails to confirm the costive habits they were intended to remove, and to disorders for life the organs of digestion. In week stomachs uric and other acids are evolved, causing gout, gravel, stiffness and concretion of the joints – the solution will always palliate and often remove those afflicting complaints. Indigestion and many disorders of the system, frequently proceed from an acidulous state of the stomach, and children are particularly subject to this depraved condition of the organ, in consequence of their existing almost exclusively on milk and vegetable diet. A small quantity of solution (which children drink with avidity and in general prefer to every other beverage) will in a short time, neutralize the existing acid, and if continued will prevent the formation of any new acid. Independent of the other advantages the solution possesses over crude Magnesia or other medicine, intends to procure similar effects. The superior purity of the Magnesia contained in the solution, (the proprietor having discovered a process by which he deprives the Magnesia he makes, use of the numerous impurities it is always contaminated with) must give it a decided preference over every other preparation. To avoid the appearance of imposition, the certificate of the Physicians and other approbatory testimonials are not published, but may be seen at the store of the subscriber.

The solution may be either drank at the fount (as mineral waters) at 12 ½ cents per half pint, or may be had in bottles of an oval shape of different sizes, marked in raised letters "Cullen's Liquid Magnesia", and labelled Cullen's Solution of Magnesia.

Observe none is genuine except what answers the above description, and is signed by the sole proprietor, **John Cullen**.

Price – large bottle $3 per doz. – small $2.

75 cents for the large, 50 for the small bottles, will be refunded on returning the empty bottles. Sold on very liberal terms to Physicians, packed in the best manner and forwarded to any part of the United States. The poor and charitable institutions supplied at ½ price.

Sold in Philadelphia (only) at Cullen's Drug and Chemical Warehouse. N.E. corner of Chestnut and Second Streets, and by his agents throughout the United States.

Mineral waters of every description. Apr 30

****

Ad number 3:

By Letters Patent From the U. States
Cullen's Patent Solution of Magnesia

For sale as usual at the Patentee's store NE corner of Chestnut & Second Streets.
May 20

****

John Cullen lowered the price of his bottled "Magnesia mineral water" several days before he added the Patent information to the 1st ad (May 7, 1818).

From April 30 through May 5 – (price $3.50 for large bottles - $2.50 for the small bottles)
From May 6 through May 19 - (price $3 for large bottles - $2 for the small bottles)
From May20 through May 26 – (price is not mentioned)
All prices (or refunds) mentioned in the ads are for a dozen bottles.

One can only wonder what other kinds of mineral waters he sold according to the last line of his 1st & 2nd advertisements ("***Mineral waters of every description***").

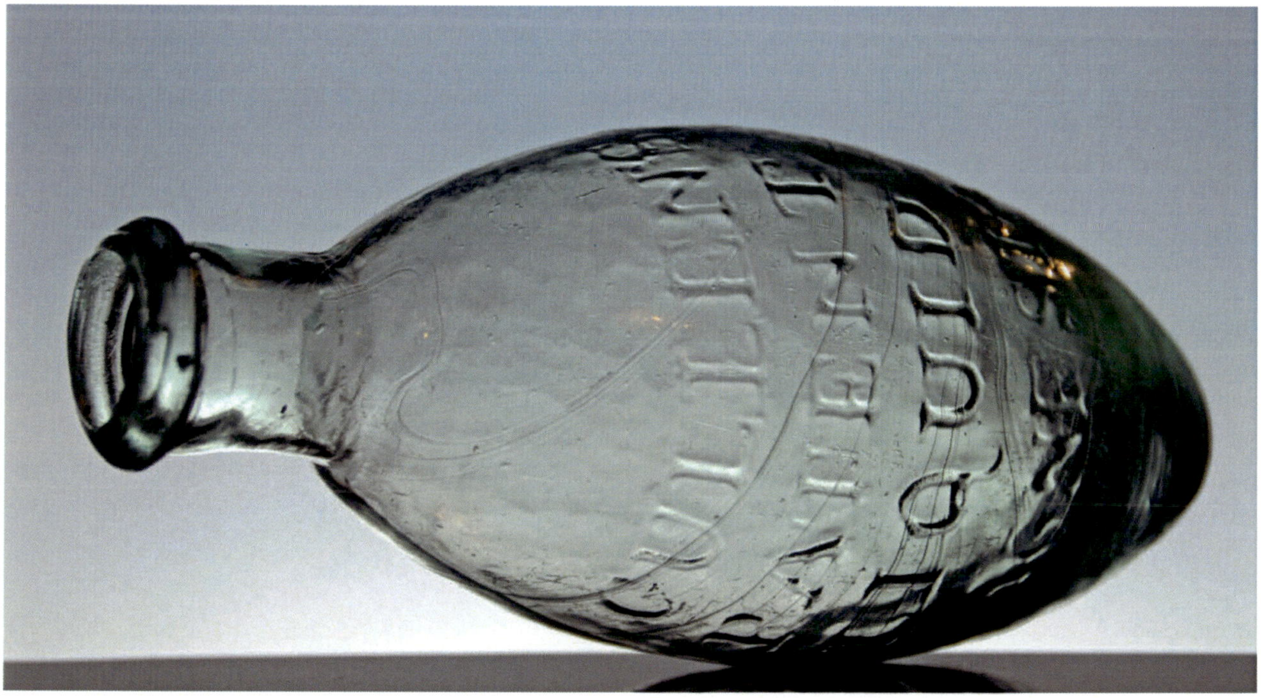

US Letter Patent Granted May 4, 1818 to John Cullen of Philadelphia

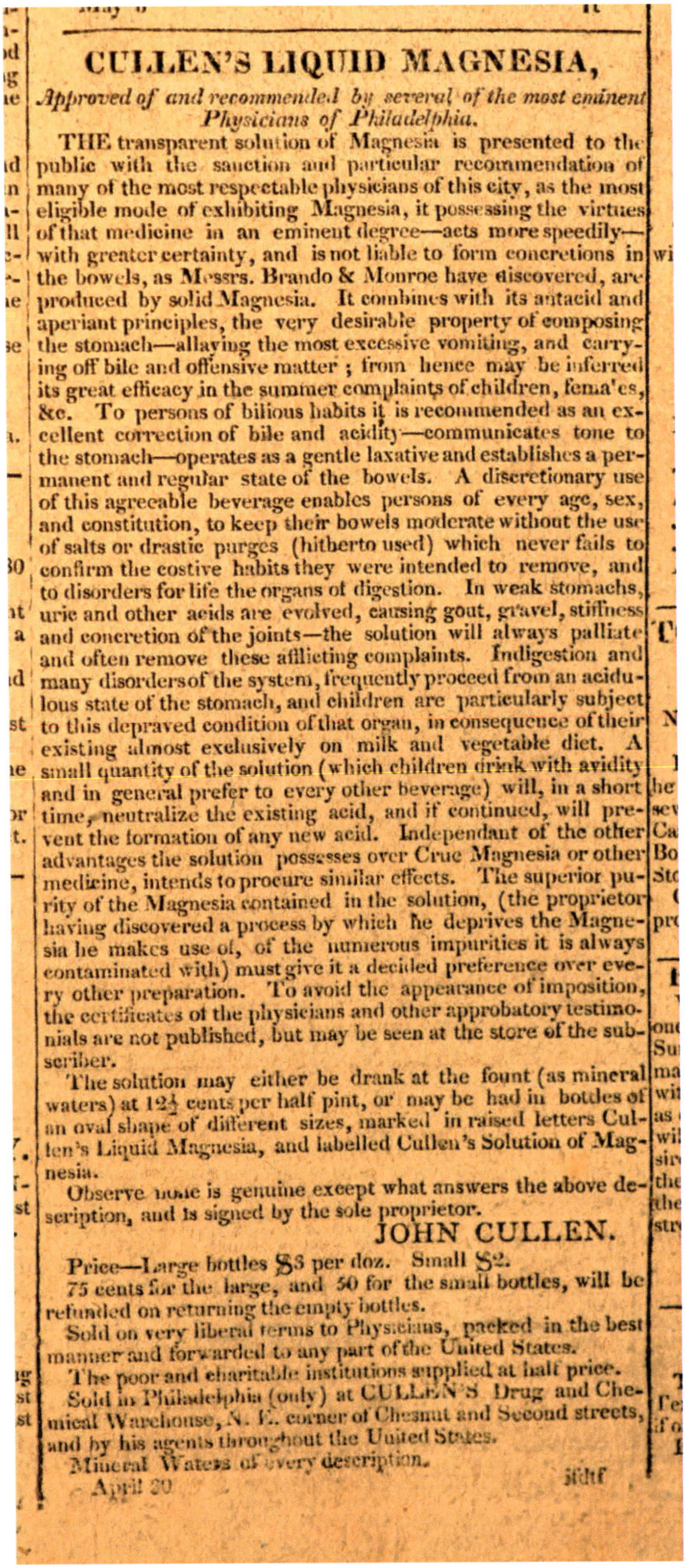

CULLEN'S LIQUID MAGNESIA,

Approved of and recommended by several of the most eminent Physicians of Philadelphia.

THE transparent solution of Magnesia is presented to the public with the sanction and particular recommendation of many of the most respectable physicians of this city, as the most eligible mode of exhibiting Magnesia, it possessing the virtues of that medicine in an eminent degree—acts more speedily—with greater certainty, and is not liable to form concretions in the bowels, as Messrs. Brando & Monroe have discovered, are produced by solid Magnesia. It combines with its antacid and aperiant principles, the very desirable property of composing the stomach—allaying the most excessive vomiting, and carrying off bile and offensive matter ; from hence may be inferred its great efficacy in the summer complaints of children, females, &c. To persons of bilious habits it is recommended as an excellent correction of bile and acidity—communicates tone to the stomach—operates as a gentle laxative and establishes a permanent and regular state of the bowels. A discretionary use of this agreeable beverage enables persons of every age, sex, and constitution, to keep their bowels moderate without the use of salts or drastic purges (hitherto used) which never fails to confirm the costive habits they were intended to remove, and to disorders for life the organs of digestion. In weak stomachs, uric and other acids are evolved, causing gout, gravel, stiffness and concretion of the joints—the solution will always palliate and often remove these afflicting complaints. Indigestion and many disorders of the system, frequently proceed from an acidulous state of the stomach, and children are particularly subject to this depraved condition of that organ, in consequence of their existing almost exclusively on milk and vegetable diet. A small quantity of the solution (which children drink with avidity and in general prefer to every other beverage) will, in a short time, neutralize the existing acid, and if continued, will prevent the formation of any new acid. Independant of the other advantages the solution possesses over Crue Magnesia or other medicine, intends to procure similar effects. The superior purity of the Magnesia contained in the solution, (the proprietor having discovered a process by which he deprives the Magnesia he makes use of, of the numerous impurities it is always contaminated with) must give it a decided preference over every other preparation. To avoid the appearance of imposition, the certificates of the physicians and other approbatory testimonials are not published, but may be seen at the store of the subscriber.

The solution may either be drank at the fount (as mineral waters) at 12½ cents per half pint, or may be had in bottles of an oval shape of different sizes, marked in raised letters Cullen's Liquid Magnesia, and labelled Cullen's Solution of Magnesia.

Observe none is genuine except what answers the above description, and is signed by the sole proprietor.

JOHN CULLEN.

Price—Large bottles $3 per doz. Small $2.

75 cents for the large, and 50 for the small bottles, will be refunded on returning the empty bottles.

Sold on very liberal terms to Physicians, packed in the best manner and forwarded to any part of the United States.

The poor and charitable institutions supplied at half price.

Sold in Philadelphia (only) at CULLEN'S Drug and Chemical Warehouse, N. E. corner of Chesnut and Second streets, and by his agents throughout the United States.

Mineral Waters of every description.

April 30 3tdtf

John Cullen's 1st ad for his Mineral Water in oval bottles (Egg Bottles in 2 sizes). It ran from: April 30 – May 6, 1818.

This image is from May 6, 1818 as it appeared in the newspaper, "Aurora General Advertiser" of Philadelphia, Pennsylvania (page 3, column 4).

It does not mention his US patent, (granted May 4, 1818 for his mineral water, "Solution of Magnesia").

Courtesy of "*The Library Company of Philadelphia*" *(Call number 4-B-3-5)*

April 27 ifmwf12t

BY LETTERS PATENT FROM THE U. STATES,

CULLEN'S LIQUID MAGNESIA,

Approved of and recommended by several of the most eminent Physicians of Philadelphia.

THE transparent solution of Magnesia is presented to the public with the sanction and particular recommendation of many of the most respectable physicians of this city, as the most eligible mode of exhibiting Magnesia. This solution possesses the virtues of that medicine in an eminent degree—acts more speedily—with greater certainty, and is not liable to form concretions in the bowels, as Messrs. Brande & Monroe have discovered, are sometimes produced by solid Magnesia. It combines with its anttacid and aperient principles, the very desirable property of composing the stomach—allaying the most excessive vomiting, and carrying off bile and offensive matter. Hence may be inferred its great efficacy in the summer complaints of children, females, &c.

To persons of bilious habits it is recommended as an excellent corrector of bile and acidity—communicates tone to the stomach—operates as a gentle laxative and establishes a permanent and regular state of the bowels.

A discretionary use of this agreeable beverage enables persons of every age, sex, and constitution, to keep their bowels moderate without the use of salts or drastic purges (hitherto used) which never fail to confirm the costive habits they were intended to remove, and to disorders for life the organs of digestion.

In weak stomachs uric and other acids are evolved, causing gout, gravel, stiffness and concretion of the joints—the solution will always palliate and often remove these afflicting complaints. *Indigestion* and many disorders of the system, frequently proceed from an acidulous state of the stomach; children are particularly subject to this depraved condition of that organ, in consequence of their existing almost exclusively on milk and vegetable diet. A small quantity of the solution (which children drink with avidity, and in general prefer to every other beverage) will, in a short time, neutralize the existing acid, and if continued, will prevent the formation of any new acid.

Independant of the other advantages the solution possesses over Crude Magnesia or any other medicine, intended to procure similar effects, the *superior purity* of the Magnesia contained in the solution, (the patentee having discovered a process by which he deprives the Magnesia he makes use of, of the numerous impurities it is always contaminated with) must give it a decided preference over every other preparation. To avoid the appearance of empiricism, the certificates of the physicians and other approbatory testimonials are not published, but may be seen at the store of the subscriber.

The solution may either be drank at the fount (as mineral waters) at 12½ cents per half pint, or may be had in bottles of an oval shape of different sizes, marked in raised letters "Cullen's Liquid Magnesia," and labelled *Cullen's Solution of Magnesia.*

Observe none is genuine except what answers the above description, and is signed by the sole proprietor.

JOHN CULLEN.

Price—Large bottles $3 per doz. Small $2.

75 cents for the large, and 50 for the small bottles, will be refunded on returning the empty bottles.

Sold on very liberal terms to Physicians, packed in the best manner and forwarded to any part of the United States.

The poor and charitable institutions supplied at half price.

Sold in Philadelphia (only) at CULLEN'S Drug and Chemical Warehouse, N. E. corner of Chesnut and Second streets, and by his agents throughout the United States.

Mineral Waters of every description.

April 30 ¶dtf

FIRST BRIGADE, FIRST DIVISION,

NINTH REGIMENT, PA. INFANTRY.

John Cullen's 2nd ad for his Mineral Water in oval bottles (Egg Bottles in 2 sizes).
May 7 – May 19, 1818.

This image is from May 11, 1818 as it appeared in the newspaper, "Aurora General Advertiser" of Philadelphia, Pennsylvania (page 3, column 4).

It now mentions his US patent, (granted May 4, 1818 for his mineral water, "Solution of Magnesia"). Spelling corrections and paragraph indentation were added as well.

Courtesy of "*The Library Company of Philadelphia*" *(Call number 4-B-3-5)*

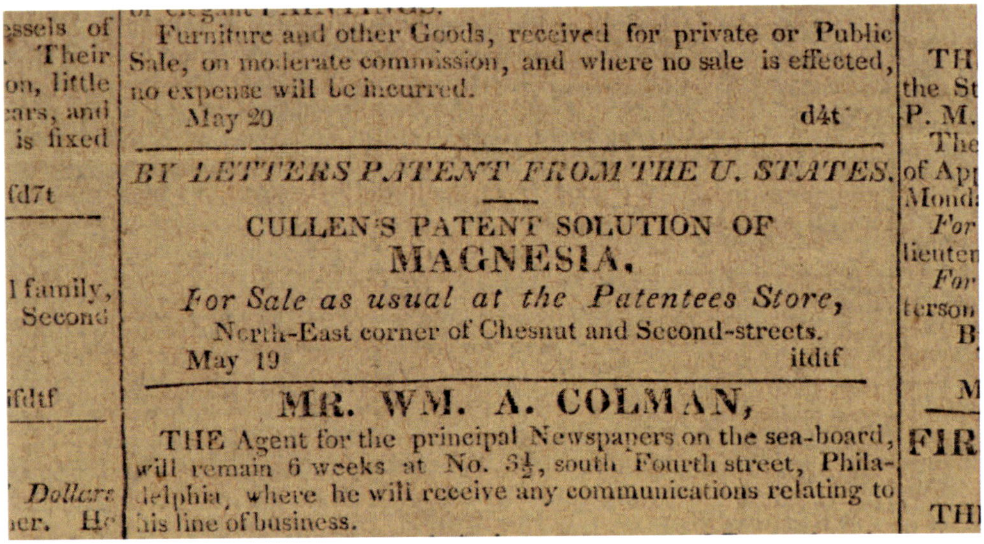

Furniture and other Goods, received for private or Public Sale, on moderate commission, and where no sale is effected, no expense will be incurred.

May 20 d4t

BY LETTERS PATENT FROM THE U. STATES.

CULLEN'S PATENT SOLUTION OF

MAGNESIA.

For Sale as usual at the Patentees Store,

North-East corner of Chesnut and Second-streets.

May 19 itdtf

MR. WM. A. COLMAN,

THE Agent for the principal Newspapers on the sea-board, will remain 6 weeks at No. 3½, south Fourth street, Philadelphia, where he will receive any communications relating to his line of business.

John Cullen's 3rd ad appeared from May 20, 1818 through May 26, 1818.

This image is from May 20, 1818 as it appeared in the newspaper, "Aurora General Advertiser" of Philadelphia, Pennsylvania (page 3, column 4). It also mentions his US patent as being for his invented "Solution of Magnesia".

Courtesy of "*The Library Company of Philadelphia*"
(Call number 4-B-3-5)

Given the authoritative level of OSD evidence listed in Appendix B, it is likely that James S. Ewing's patented (1817) mineral water manufacturing equipment was what allowed John Cullen to load his light weight glass egg bottles. Up to this time, no commercial level packaging of light weight glass "*soda water*" bottles had been possible because of the danger of explosion. Cullen is likely the very first at a commercial level - beyond the experimental.

Next to follow at the commercial level, was *Elias Durand* who started using embossed light weight bottles for mineral water after 1825. His artifacts (*see page 64*) were cylinder in shape. The need for an egg shape proved unnecessary with the safety of Ewing's mineral water manufacturing equipment.

A second generation followed in the late 1830's and early 1840's. These bottlers can easily be identified because they continued using the words "*Patent*" and "*Patent Improved*" to identify their individual mineral water and manufacturing processes, (i.e. "*double pressure*" etc.) - following John Cullen's lead of 1818.

These bottles are all of the light weight type and all were produced during the open pontil and scar pontil era of the late 1830's and early 1840's, (before the improved pontil came into general use in glasshouses in mid 1840's).

Some of this next generation of Philadelphia mineral water bottlers who continued using "*Patent*" (just as John Cullen had in 1818), includes: *William Heiss Jr., Eugene Roussel, David Bentley, John Diehl, R. Flanagan, Peter Hall, Dr. Hartley, C.Jones, etc.*. This was done in other American cities as well. Of course, the patent office fire of 1836 which caused the US Congress to rescind all previous patents was likely the motivating factor in the usage of "Patent" embossed in their bottles. As most rushed to claim patents for anything that was previously patented - probably believing a business advantage was being achieved by their deception.

The practice of claiming false "Patents" was short lived however. It was discontinued after 1844, although a few examples pop up later, mostly related to glass manufacturing patents or bottle closure design patents. These later "Patents" were validly obtained as opposed to the majority of "Patents" dubiously claimed in the period between 1837 and 1844.

Let's return to the era of our egg bottle (1818). The archaeological record confirms that no other similar artifacts have been discovered earlier than Cullen's glass bottles in the US (and possibly England as well). With James Ewing's business address on Chestnut Street (from years 1813-1825), only a few blocks from John Cullen's on Chestnut Street (from years 1818–1819), Cullen likely knew Ewing, just as well as he did Thomas W. Dyott, (the maker of his bottles).

In 1818, with the most advanced mineral water manufacturing equipment in the world available just a few blocks away, John Cullen must have recognized a ready market was at his finger tips for bottling artificial soda water. His friendships included some of the most influential Philadelphia physicians of that time, "*Dr. Physick, Dr Dorsey. Dr. Coxe, etc.*", and he had ready outlets including his own drug store and the Philadelphia Alms house.

John Cullen's egg bottle is likely at the very beginning, if not the very first, of the traditional embossed "*soda pop*" bottles. In a chain reaction, this group of Philadelphia pioneers started, what has grown into the massive industry we know today. These "*Chestnut Street*" entrepreneurs built upon each other and their improvements spread outward across regions and continents.

At the time of John Cullen's newspaper ads, in 1818, he was only 22 years old and already a US patent holder. As owner of an end to end business enterprise built solely by his own hard work he was a rarity, even by today's fast paced standards. Seldom is such accomplished without a substantial family inheritance forming the foundation. To imagine that John was also a full time medical student at the same time and donating his time to the Philadelphia Almshouse too - is incredible. His potential business success was clearly cut short due to the death of his dear friend, Dr. John Syng Dorsey and his move to Virginia.

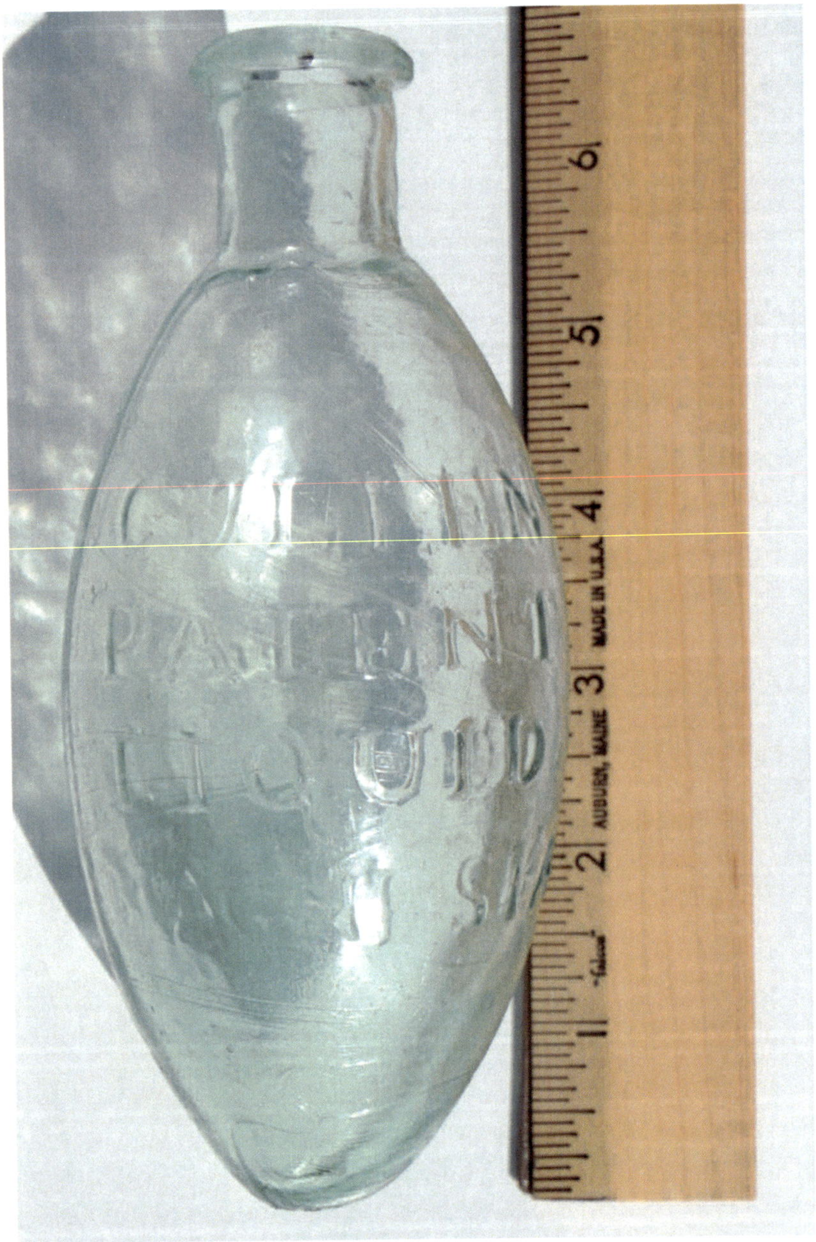

An archaeological reference picture - Color is slightly lighter than normal.
Earliest known marked artificial mineral water bottle in American history (1818)
(Size - 6 1/8 in high by 2 11/16 in diameter at the center)

Sample artifacts in the Evolution of the US egg bottle (1830-1845)

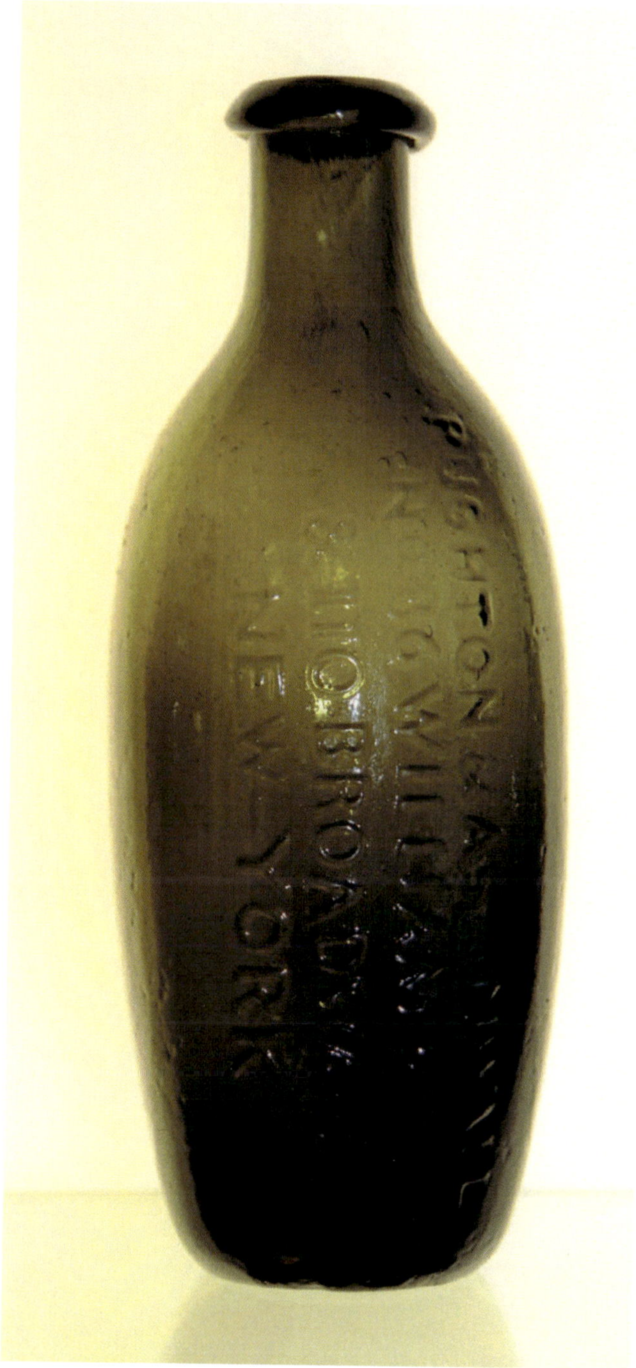

Rushton & Aspinwall / No 86 William St / & 110 Broadway / New York
(William L Rushton & James S. Aspinwall - Druggists)
Artifact circa 1833 – 1837 – sand pontil
Courtesy of "*Dr. Eric L. Schmetterling*"

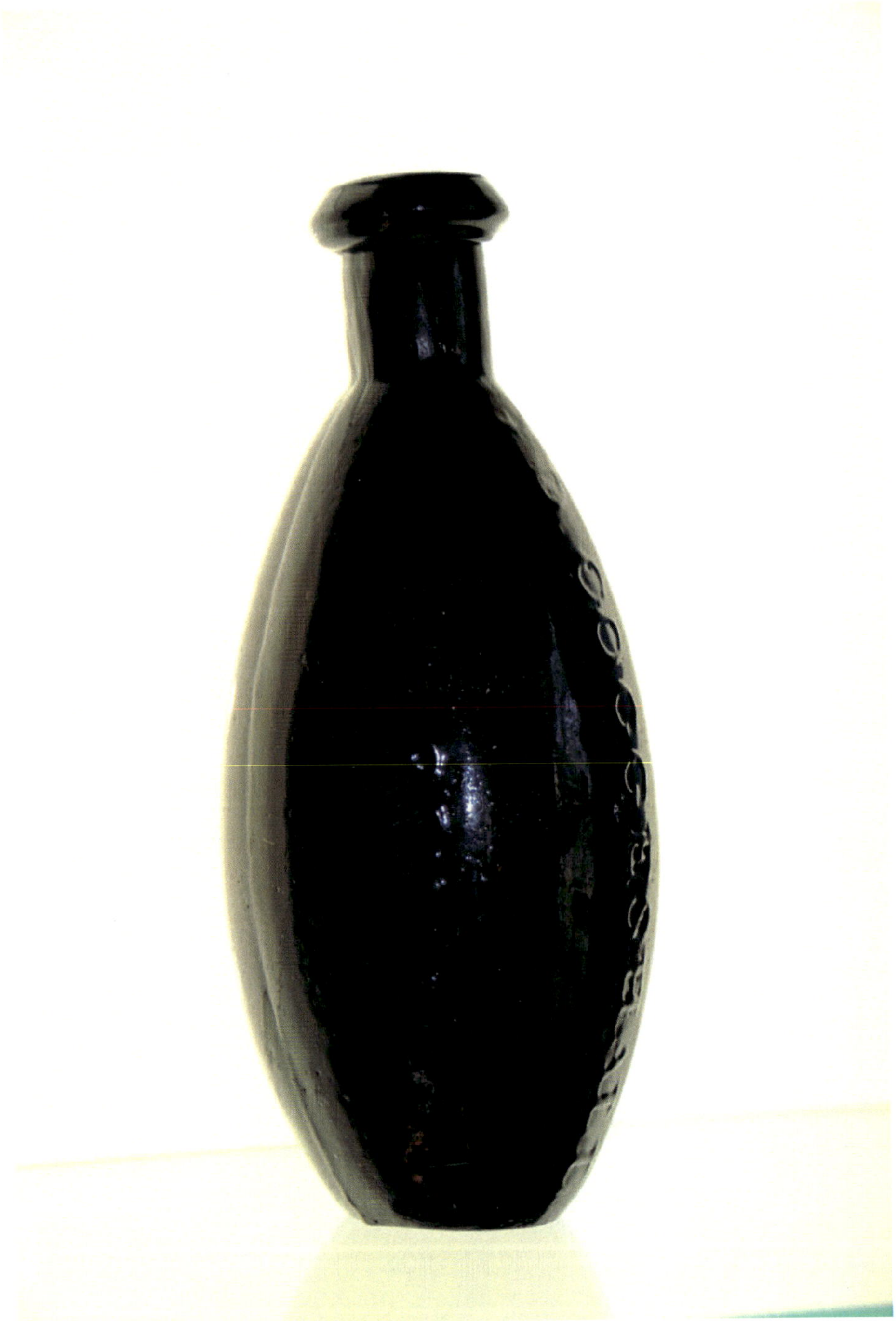

G.D. Coggeshall / 421 Pearl St. / New York / Soda Water
(View 1) George D. Coggeshall – Druggist)
Artifact circa 1830 – 1837 – sand pontil
Courtesy of "*Dr. Eric L. Schmetterling*"

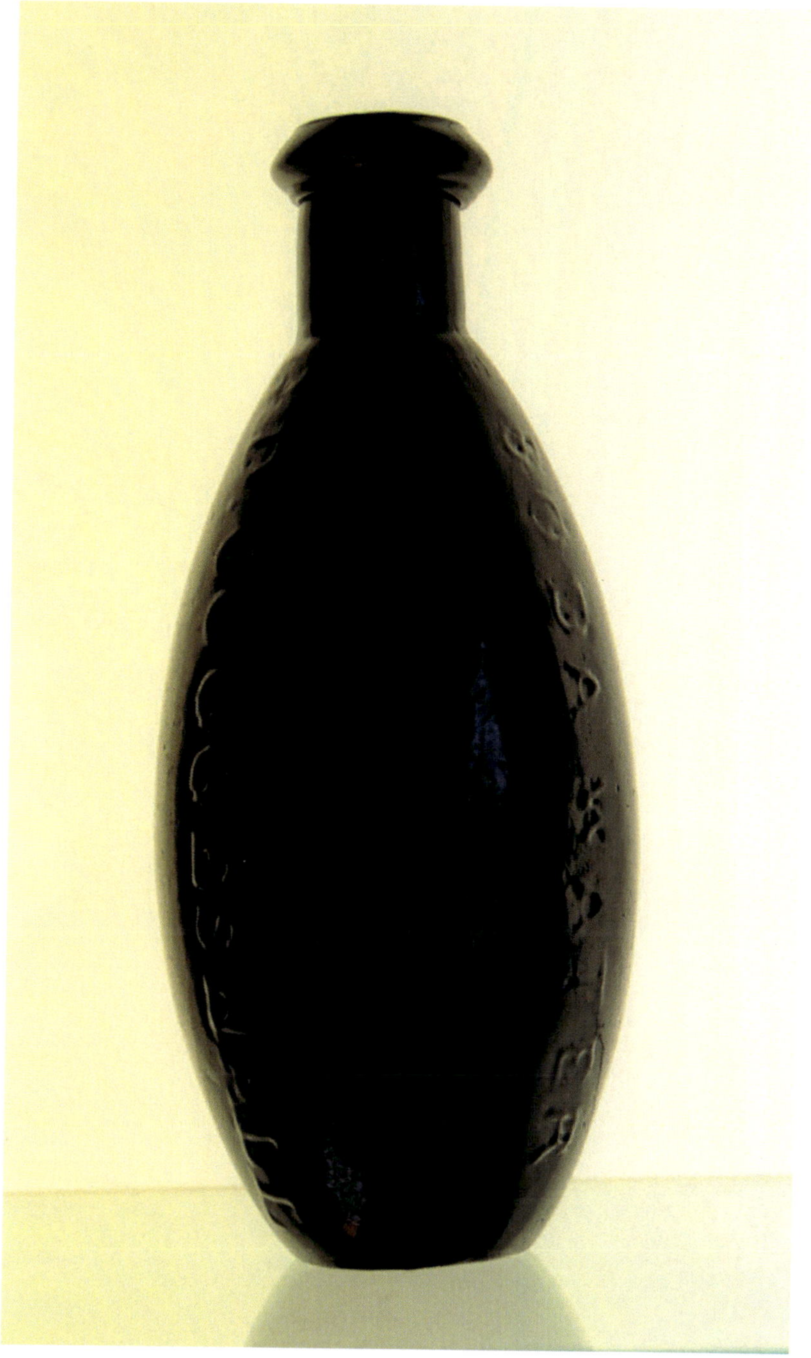

G.D. Coggeshall / 421 Pearl St. / New York / Soda Water
(View 2) (George D. Coggeshall – Druggist)
Artifact circa 1830 – 1837 – sand pontil
Courtesy of "*Dr. Eric L. Schmetterling*"

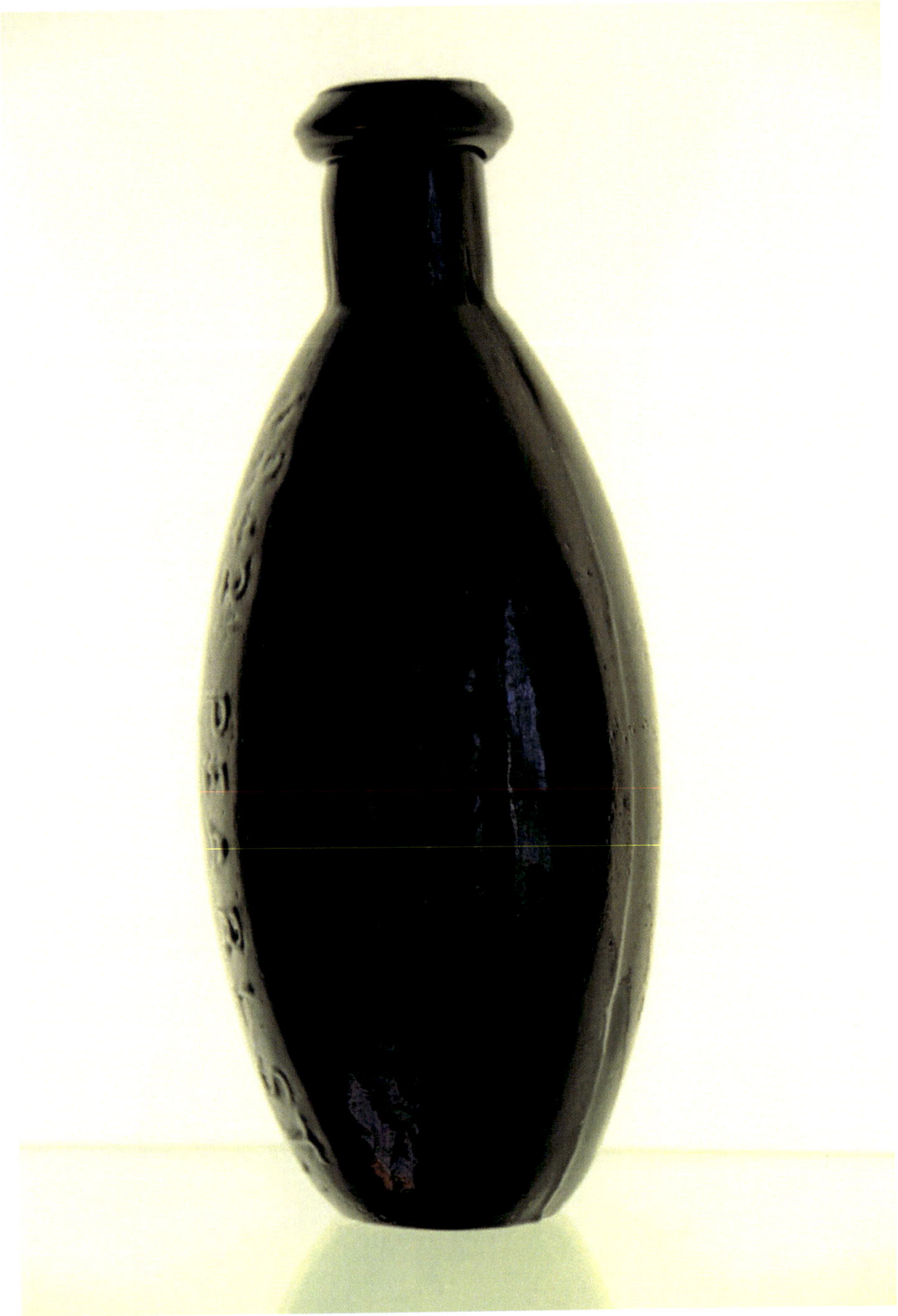

G.D. Coggeshall / 421 Pearl St. / New York / Soda Water
(View 3) (George D. Coggeshall – Druggist)
Artifact circa 1830 – 1837 – sand pontil
Courtesy of "*Dr. Eric L. Schmetterling*"

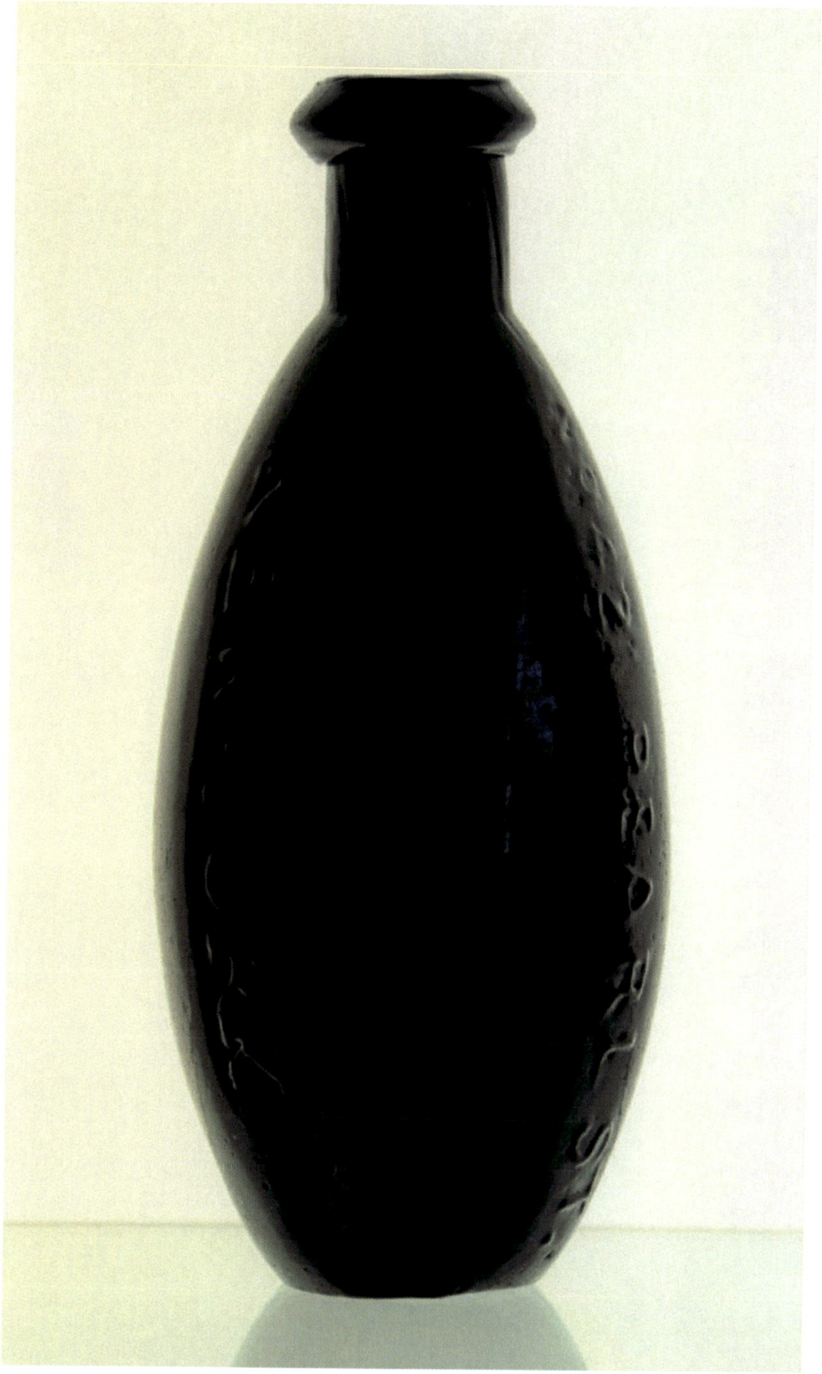

G.D. Coggeshall / 421 Pearl St. / New York / Soda Water
(View 4) (George D. Coggeshall – Druggist)
Artifact circa 1830 – 1837 – sand pontil
Courtesy of "*Dr. Eric L. Schmetterling*"

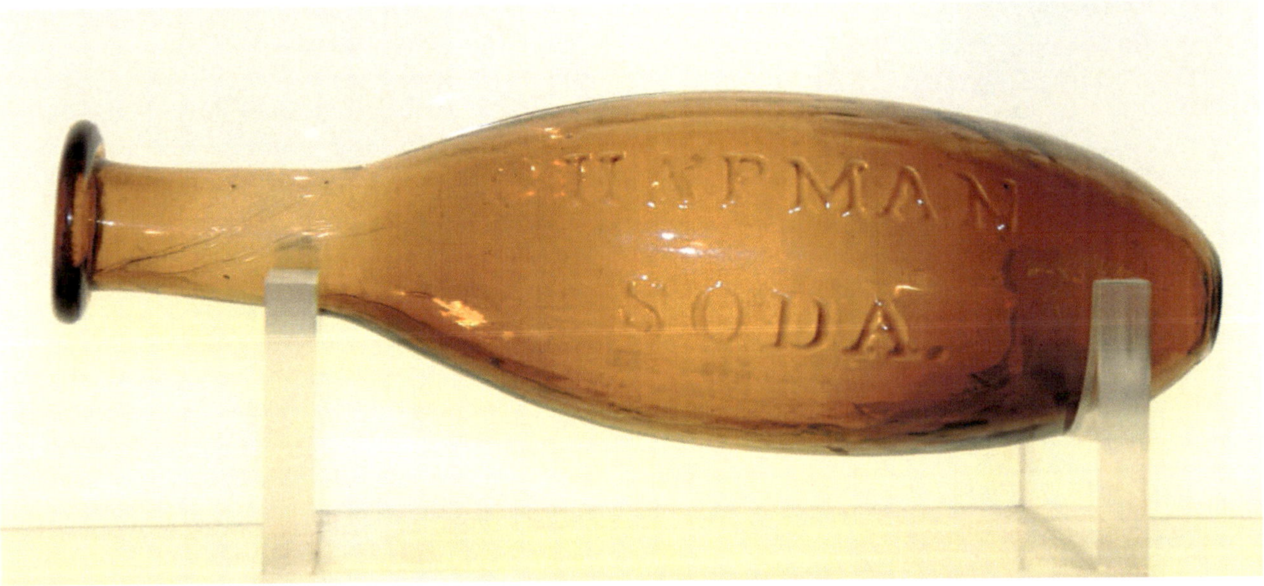

Chapman / Soda
Baltimore, Maryland
Artifact circa 1835-1845 – no pontil
Courtesy of "*Dr. Eric L. Schmetterling*"

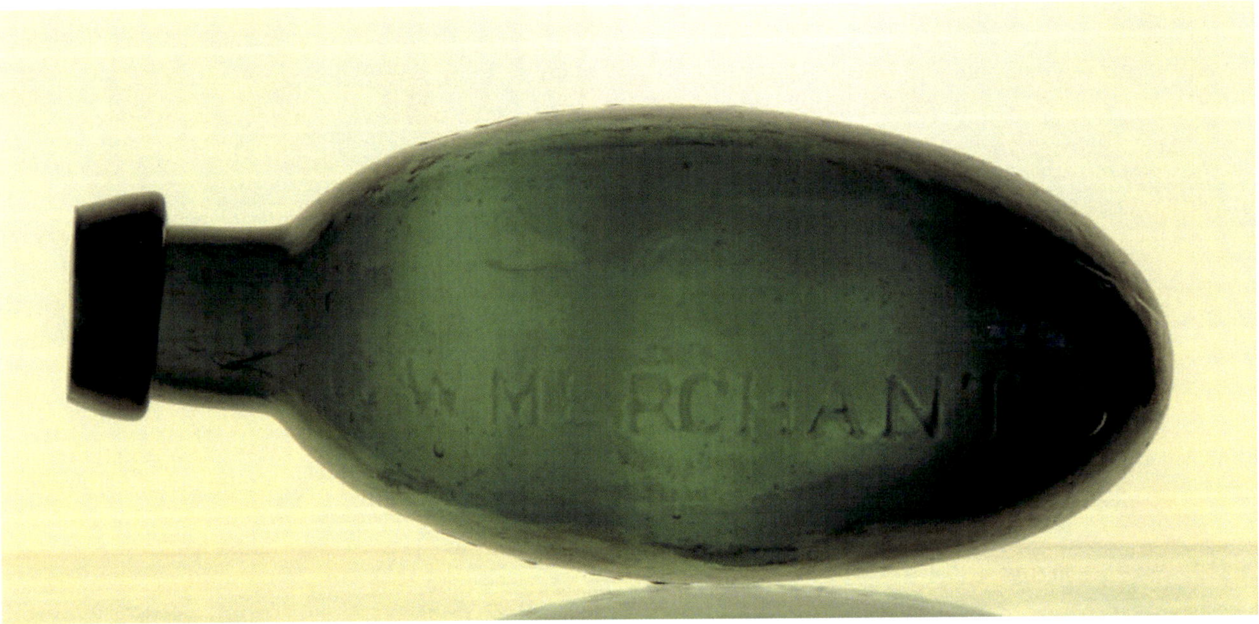

G. W. Merchant / Carbonic / Mineral Water / Lockport NY
(View 1) (George W. Merchant – Chemist & Pharmaceutist)
Artifact circa 1845 – no pontil
Courtesy of "*Dr. Eric L. Schmetterling*"

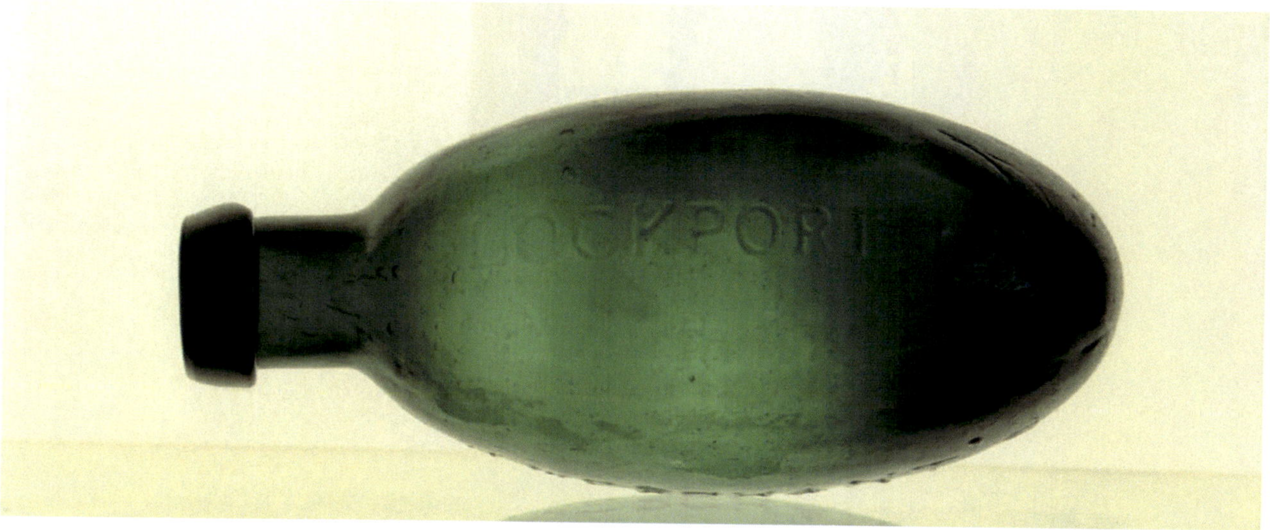

G. W. Merchant / Carbonic / Mineral Water / Lockport NY
(View 2) (George W. Merchant – Chemist & Pharmaceutist)
Artifact circa 1845 – no pontil
Courtesy of "*Dr. Eric L. Schmetterling*"

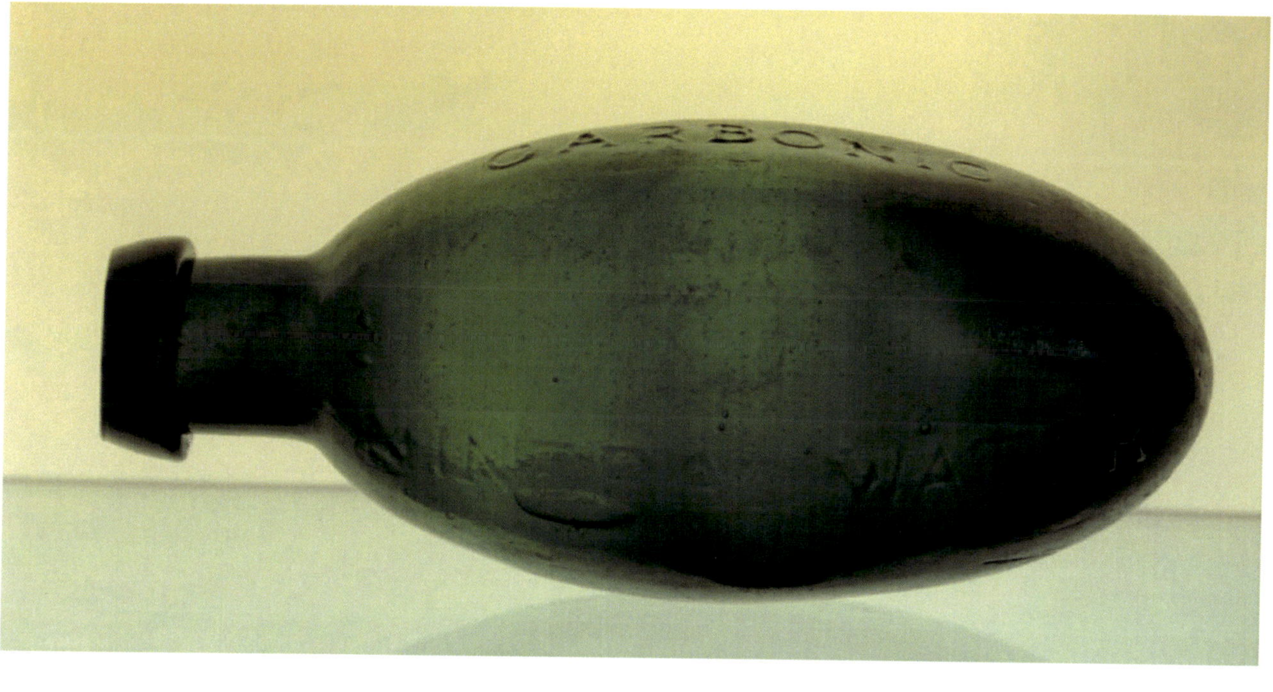

G. W. Merchant / Carbonic / Mineral Water / Lockport NY
(View 3) (George W. Merchant – Chemist & Pharmaceutist)
Artifact circa 1845 – no pontil
Courtesy of "*Dr. Eric L. Schmetterling*"

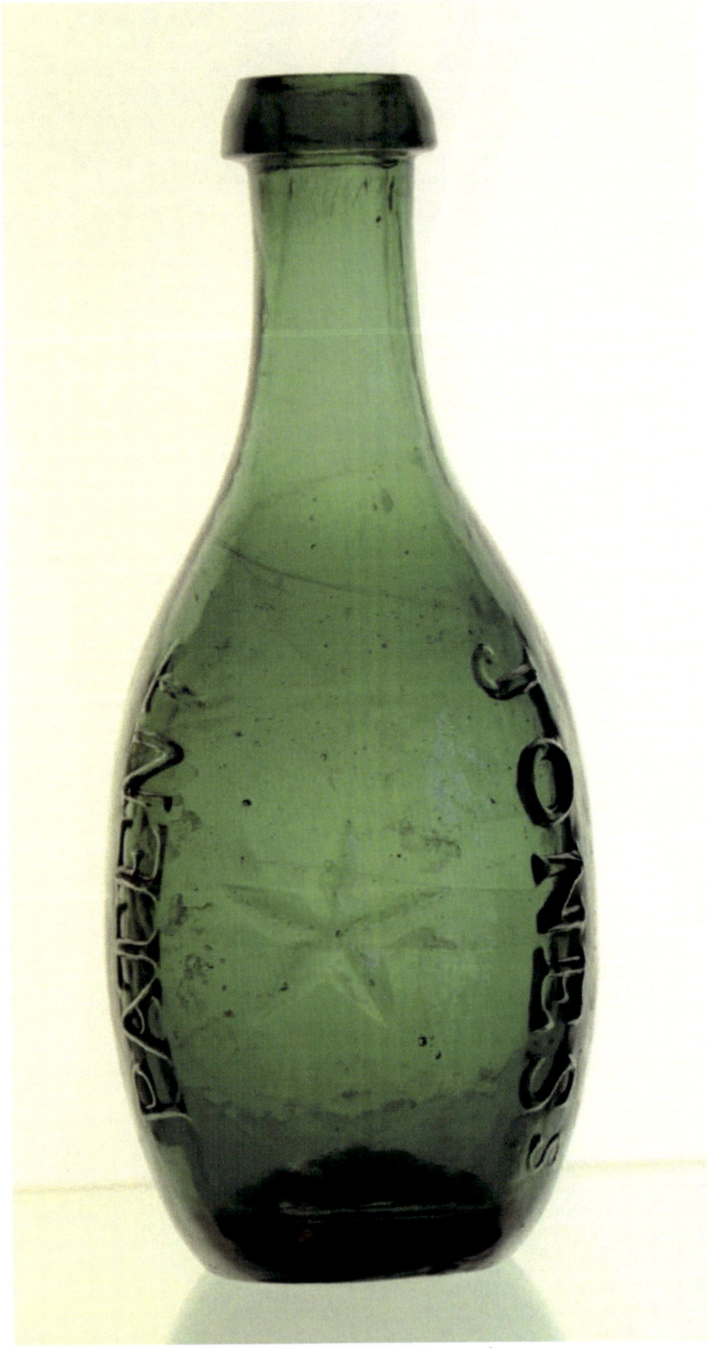

Jones's / Patent / Mineral / Water
(View 1) (Cornelius Jones - Philadelphia – Tavern Owner)
Artifact circa 1844-1845 – Improved pontil (i.e. *Iron Pontil*)
Courtesy of "*Dr. Eric L. Schmetterling*"

Jones is one of those who belong to the dubious club of questionable patent claim holders following the Washington DC patent office fire of December 1836. It is likely whatever patent was claimed, was copied from some previous patent that was burned and then rescinded by Congress in 1837. Jones later dropped this claim. Embossing "Patent" in raised letters on mineral water bottles clearly started with John Cullen.

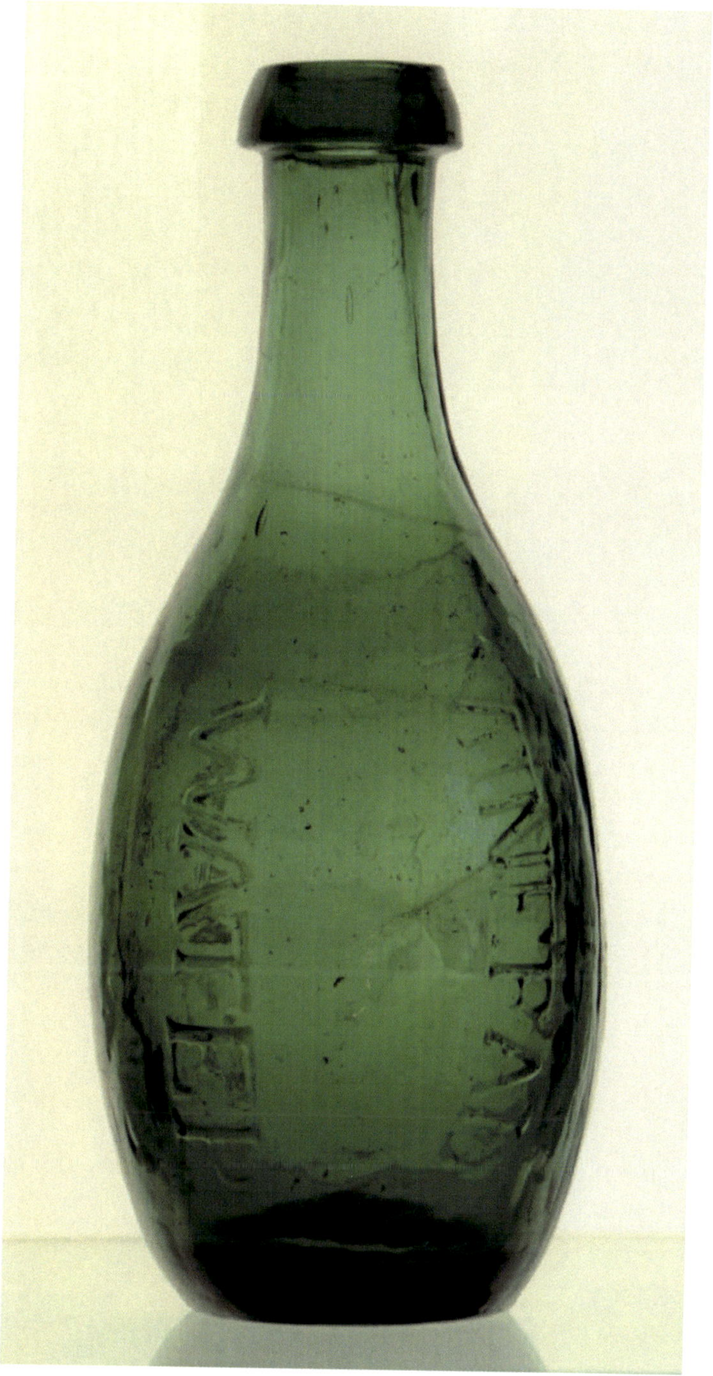

Jones's / Patent / Mineral / Water
(View 2) (Cornelius Jones - Philadelphia – Tavern Owner)
Artifact circa 1844-1845 – Improved pontil (i.e. *Iron Pontil*)
Courtesy of "*Dr. Eric L. Schmetterling*"

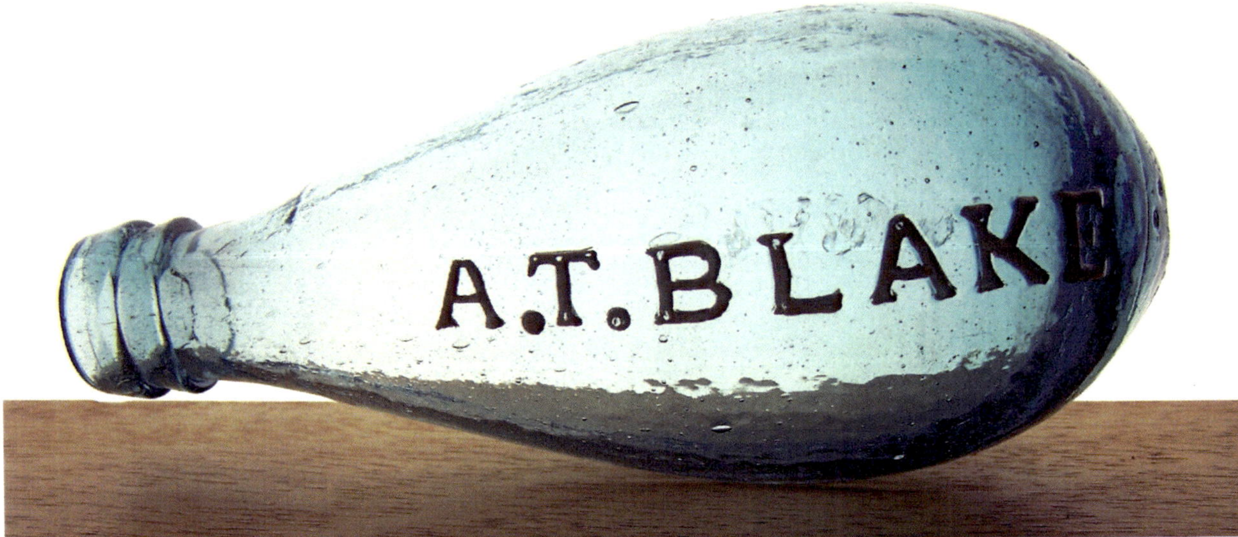

A. T. Blake / Cincinnati
(View 1) (Alexander T. Blake – Druggist)
Artifact circa 1838 -1841 – open ring pontil – small flat base
Courtesy of "*Jim Hall*"

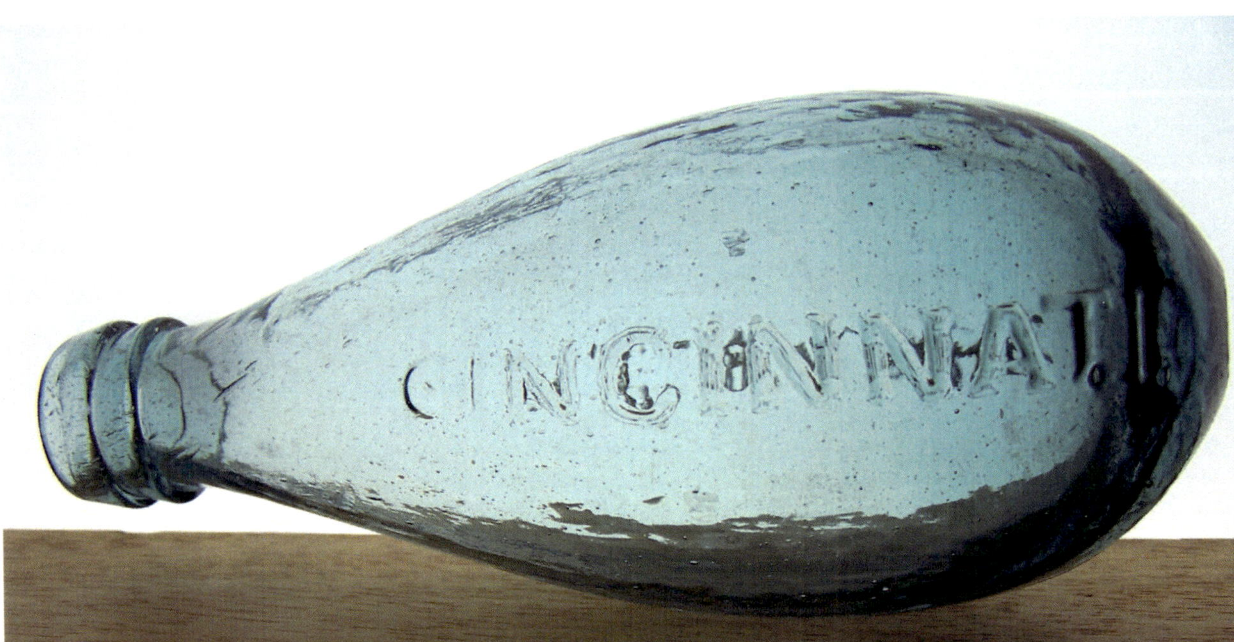

A. T. Blake / Cincinnati
(View 2) Courtesy of "*Jim Hall*"

One of the more unusual egg bottles is A.T. Blake from Cincinnati, Ohio. It has a rare double collar top and light bulb shape. It is likely one of the last open pontilled egg bottles. Alexander Blake was listed as a druggist at Burdsal's Drug Store from 1839 to 1840. By 1842 he is no longer listed. In 1846 he re-appears as a feather dealer.

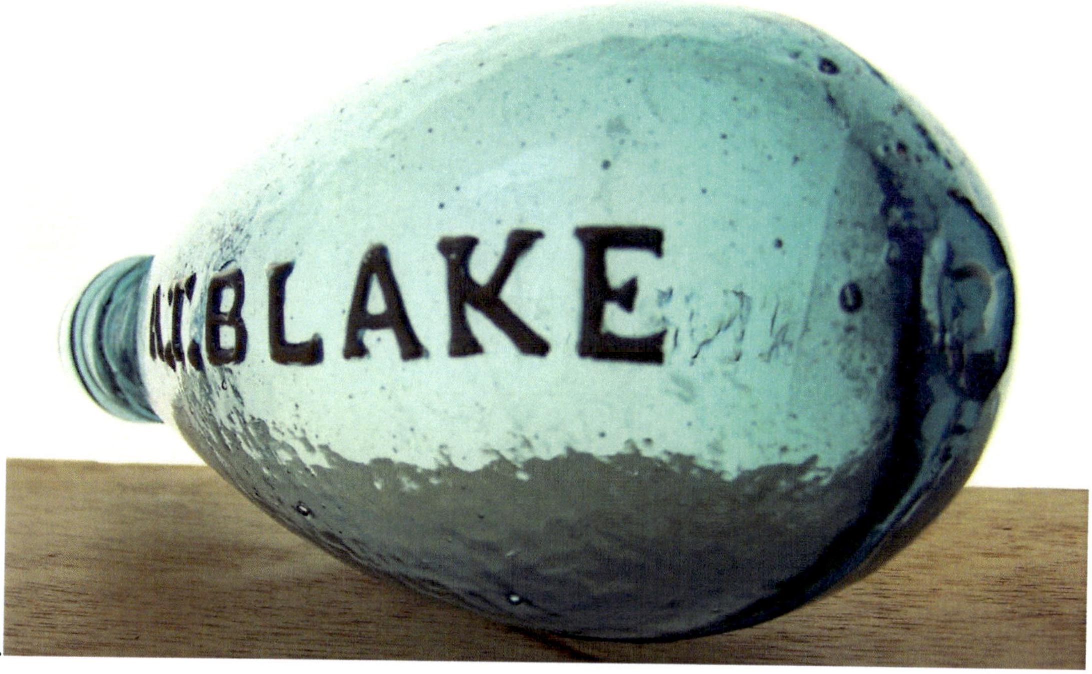

A. T. Blake / Cincinnati
(View 3) Courtesy of "*Jim Hall*"

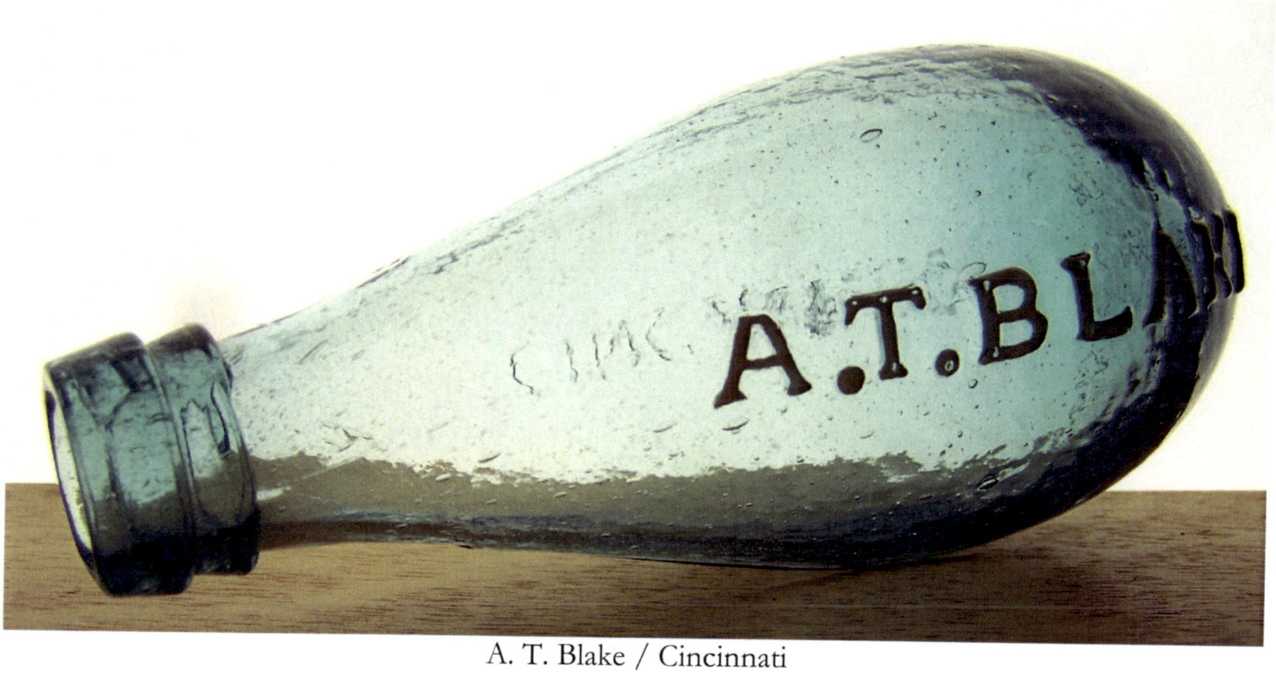

A. T. Blake / Cincinnati
(View 4) Courtesy of "*Jim Hall*"

Shaffer's Advertising Directory, Cincinnati Ohio in 1839 and 1840 adds the abbreviation "*Eng*" to Blake's occupation as a "*Druggist*". This may indicate "engineer". Many early mineral water bottlers considered themselves to be engineers as they often constructed their own bottling equipment and plumbing for drugstore soda fountains.

6 The Web of Characters and Events - *(Timeline)*

John Cullen

Age	Timeline Events *(Chronology)*
0	Born Dublin Ireland (about) February 2,1796 (Possibly son of *Erin Cullen*)
17-18	Attends Trinity College – natural sciences, classics, and chemistry – 1813-1814
18	Visits Paris France - 1814
18-19	Prisoner of *Napoleon*, then paroled – Paris France – 1814 / 1815
19	Battle of Waterloo won by *Wellington* and "Coalition Forces" – June 18, 1815
19	Returns to England with the "Allied Sovereigns" upon their visit – July 1815
19	Emigrates to America - arriving in New York City on September 29, 1815
20	Enters University of Pennsylvania Medical School – 1816
21	Begins work at Philadelphia Alms House (volunteer work?) – June 1817
21	Becomes a "Naturalized" American citizen in Philadelphia. October 28, 1817
22	First Listed in Philadelphia Directory as Chymist and Druggist – 1818
22	First newspaper ad started (*Aurora General Advertiser*) – April 30, 1818 First ad listing an "*embossed*" mineral water glass bottle, that actually exists First ad listing an "*oval*" egg glass bottle of US origin, that actually exists
22	Awarded Letter Patent from US for "Liquid Magnesia" – May 4, 1818 First United States Patent for soda water (*artificial mineral water*)
22	Second newspaper ad started (Aurora) – May 7, 1818 to May 19, 1818
22	Third newspaper ad started – May 20, 1818 to May 26, 1818
22	*John Syng Dorsey* passes away at 35 years of age – November 1818
22	*John Cullen* writes letter to U of P requesting MD degree – December 28, 1818
23	*Thomas W. Dyott* begins listing "Liquid Magnesia bottles" for sale - 1819
23	Receives MD degree from U of P – April 15, 1819
23	Last year Philadelphia Dir. lists drugstore (NE cor. 2nd & Chestnut) - 1819
24	Philadelphia Directory lists occupation as doctor (new address) – 1820
24	May have become Philadelphia Alms House Physician? - 1820
24-25	*Thomas Jefferson* invites John Cullen to visit the University of Virginia –1820/21
24-25	Becomes ill in Virginia and recovers in Richmond – 1820/21
26	Last Philadelphia directory listing for *John Cullen* MD – 1822
28	Hand written Medical Bill by John Cullen from Richmond, Va. – 1824
31/32	Marries *Charlotte Howard* (2 sons & 2 daughters)? (1827 or February 28,1828)
36	Son is born,"*John Syng Dorsey Cullen*" July 29,1832 (who becomes MD as well)
42	One of the founders of "*Medical College of Virginia*" (today VCU) – 1838
26-53	Teaches and/or practices medicine in Richmond – 1822 through 1849
48-50	*Charlotte Howard Cullen* complains to MCV chancellor about John – 1844-1846
52-53	Philadelphia Drug firm starts marketing "*Cullen's Remedies*" – 1848 / 49
53	Passes away – Dec 25, 1849
53	Buried in Richmond, Virginia, (Hollywood Cemetery)

Known Significant Associations in the Timeline

- Napoleon Bonaparte,
- *President* Thomas Jefferson,
- *Dr.* Thomas W. Dyott,
- *Dr.* John Syng Dorsey,
- *Dr.* John Redman Coxe,
- Hampden–Sydney College / Medical College of Va. (*Va. Commonwealth Unv.*)
- University of Pennsylvania
- *Dr.* John Syng Dorsey Cullen (son of John Cullen)
- Rowand & Walton, Philadelphia Commercial Druggists

Likely, Significant Associations in the Timeline

- James S Ewing

7 So what is the Big Deal?

- *First marked mineral water bottle in US.*
- *First marked glass bottle with a US patent embossed on it.*
- *Thought only to be of foreign manufacture in 1818 – (egg bottles).*
- *Not believed made until mid 1830's – since known US egg bottles, all have attached tops.*
- *Sheared lip with narrow string ring below lip – likely unknown in this type of bottle.*
- *Domestic manufacture T. W. Dyott (Olive, Gloucester, or Kensington glassworks).*
- *John Cullen's US X patent that has not been reconstructed - until now.*
- *Extremely early usage period and range – mid 1818.*
- *Chestnut Street is likely birthplace that started our current soda water industry.*
- *Backed by direct historical record descriptions of the bottle, contents, and patent.*
- *Bottle existed in two (2) sizes (large & small) – first evidence of multiple sizes.*
- *Liquid Magnesia bottles were a regular glassware product carried in T.W.Dyott's national catalogue (see 1820 Dyott catalogue).*
- *The consolidated tale of John Cullen and his tremendous accomplishments.*
- *Reconstruction of 3 more US X Patents that had not been reconstructed - until now. Joseph Hawkins (1 patent), James S. Ewing (2 patents), (see Appendix B).*
- *The story of James S Ewing and his explosion proof mineral water equipment.*

The story of the egg bottle (artifact) has acquired so much more - perspective and illumination - perhaps "*national treasure*" status.

One must wonder, would the tale of John Cullen have been lost in time, but for this lone artifact showing us how to remember?

Such a new story rarely unfolds in the quiet of the academic world. Because historians and researchers have the tale sketched out already. Occasionally the archaeologist can illuminate the academic story whereby the tale is confirmed or modified. Here the tale is written anew. That is what raises it to spectacular heights.

Certainly the artifacts are rare, possibly unique. Duplicate artifacts may exist and merely passed over by my peers due to other areas of interest to them. My peers and others will surely build upon my shoulders as I have theirs, in so many other areas of research and discovery.

John Cullen's tale represents a new foundational building block for my peers, and therefore the tale itself, is a big deal.

8 Evolving Theories and Conclusion

- *Egg bottles were produced domestically.*
- *Egg bottles were produced by Thomas W..Dyott.*
- *Egg bottles were a regular catalogue item carried by T. W.Dyott.*
- *John Cullen was issued the first US patent for artificial mineral water.*
- *All mineral water related patents prior to 1818, were for mineral water fountains, manufacturing equipment, and equipment improvements.*
- *Elias Durand was not the origin of Mineral Water bottling in Philadelphia.*
- *Joseph Hawkins did not have the first patent for "artificial mineral water".*
- *A combination of individuals originated the mineral water / soda water industry in Philadelphia, including T. W.Dyott, John Cullen, Elias Durand, and James S Ewing between 1817 and 1825.*
- *Early Philadelphia pioneers from 1790 through 1812 failed to ignite the artificial mineral water and soda water industry, including commercial sized ventures by Abraham H. Cohen and George Shaw, although they tried very hard.*
- *The scarcity of egg bottles is likely due to the liberal return policy for the empties. One quarter of the original price was refunded when returned.*
- *John Matthews is not the father of the American Soda Fountain, Joseph Hawkins is by US patent.*
- *Eugene Roussel is not the father of "flavoring mineral water with sweet syrups".*
- *Embossed "Patent" and "Patent Improved" mineral water bottles from 1837 through 1844 were the result of the US Patent Office fire of 1836 and the rescinding of all US Patents prior to the fire by the US Congress (unless reconstructed). Most of these new patents were a deceptive mad rush to re-patent previous patents nullified by the government.*

Conclusion:

Based on overwhelming evidence discussed in the preceding chapters, Cullen's egg bottle is the oldest known marked mineral water bottle in the United States and may be in England as well. Without a doubt its archaeological and historical context raises it to the status of a United States treasure.

Although John Cullen's life revolved around his beloved medical college in Richmond Virginia, it is ironic that he likely never suspected his richest historic legacy would be his business interests abandoned so long ago in Philadelphia. I suspect John would be pleased to see the vast global empire that has grown from the roots of pre-1820 Philadelphia.

9

Illumination

Although Richmond Virginia has a considerable claim to John Cullen, we find Philadelphia may have just as strong a claim. Historically, the importance of his contributions in both locations has expanded as time has passed. Certainly the "*full historic*" tale is still evolving in both regions and globally as well.

John Cullen's "*patent*" was for an actual product – not just part of a process or manufacturing improvement or fountain invention (see Joseph Hawkins - Appendix B). Cullen's artificial mineral water was patented, manufactured, and marketed – a complete end to end process and product. Such illumination is shown by the archaeological artifact (oval egg bottle). Secondly it was being marketed from a soda fountain as well as being bottled as shown by historical records (original source documents – our grains of truth).

So far as historical records show, no patent was issued to anyone prior to John Cullen for "*artificial mineral water*" itself. The broad assumptions my peers have made crediting Joseph Hawkins with the first US "*artificial mineral water*" patent are clearly incorrect based on Joseph Hawkins's own advertisement in the Baltimore Whig newspaper on July 17, 1810 where he claims to hold a patent for mineral water fountain inventions and improvements. Since at that time he had only one mineral water related US patent (September 7, 1809), it is unlikely he ever held a patent for "*artificial mineral water*", although he claimed to be making artificial, "*Seltzer, Ballston, and Soda waters*".

This would make Joseph Hawkins one of the many early pioneers, but not the first. Hawkins followed many others in England and the US. The US patent office likely knew this as well. By way of illustration, in the Baltimore Whig newspaper starting on June 27, 1810 is another advertisement for essentially the same thing as Hawkins by a competitor. The ad is originally run on the front page by Abraham H. Cohen where he claims to have been making artificial mineral waters since 1808 in Philadelphia. Directories confirm his claim - listing him as "*manufacturer of artificial mineral water*" from 1809 through 1811 at 100 S 2nd Street, Philadelphia. In Cohen's *Baltimore Whig* newspaper ads of 1810 he lists a satellite manufacturing location at 21 Water Street, Baltimore Md. Cohen, like Hawkins, had no patent for "*artificial mineral water*".

In London, England, Jacob Schweppe was doing the same since at least 1792. Like Cohen and others in America, no patent was granted to Schweppe for inventing "*mineral water*".

David Grant and William Hamilton were making "*artificial mineral water*" in the early years of 19th century London and like

Hawkins in America, had obtained patents involving "*artificial mineral water*". But also, like Hawkins, each patent was for a manufacturing or fountain improvement, not the mineral water itself.

Other early 19th century English pioneers, *Joseph Bramah, William Russell, and Nicholas Paul,* made extensive written claims involving mineral water manufacturing equipment and improvements – not the mineral water itself. (*Appendix C*)

In the "*Philadelphia Medical Museum*" of 1809, pages 161–165, (an annual medical publication, 1806-1811), Dr. Richard Green publicly describes, a method of preparing artificial Cheltenham soda water highly impregnated with carbonic acid. The President of the Royal Medical Society of Edinburgh expresses the observation at the end of the article that he doubts it is an original idea.

Whether or not others were doing the same thing before John Cullen is irrelevant, because they failed to obtain a patent. The patent offices in England and the US are not allowed to grant patents for commonly held knowledge, it must be new and novel – an invention. It must be presumed John Cullen's application for patent was scrutinized on this basis, the same as all other applications are.

There is no evidence whatsoever that Hawkins was part of a larger expansion of "*artificial mineral water*" production in Baltimore or anywhere else. He obviously continues to try, but ultimately did not succeed. Even if Hawkins had partners at various times it would not have been sufficient to ignite the artificial mineral water industry because the talents would not have included all the skills necessary (i.e. plumber, glass manufacturer, chemist, marketer, etc.)

For the reasons mentioned previously in this book, it took a particular combination of different skills in close proximity, to start a type of chain reaction and that is what led to our present soda water industry today.

Hawkins's US patents were not reconstructed and broad assumptions based on a few words in a patent index, should not have been made by my peers (crediting Hawkins as having the first patent for "*artificial mineral water*" – which is a mistaken conclusion). Extensive assumptions must include the wider picture - all of the historical and archaeological records available.
(*See Appendix B*)

If we widen the Philadelphia picture further, to now include John Cullen's general location on Chestnut Street and probable associations with others nearby that are involved, or soon to be involved, on a commercial scale in the same industry, (Dyott, Ewing, Durand, etc.) - a beautiful regional pattern emerges. The pattern is in the form of a "*chain reaction*" leading to the soda water industry we have today.

Illumination!

10

Full-historic Perspective

Combined with other artifact rich tales, the broader perspective emerges from the mists of time - largely unknown. Of course the story of its general effects - spreading regionally, nationally and globally - was obvious for a long time. The origins however, of these broader cultural changes, have remained shrouded in mystery.

A subject of much speculation by researchers and historians has been the origins of our modern sugar based diet and what society needs to do to reverse some of its effects. Many school districts in the country have identified soda pop as a primary source of obesity because of the sugars contained in them. School district regulations and laws have been enacted removing these products from many of our schools.

Clearly this had its origins in the long ago patents and products of early artificial mineral water developers. For instance Abraham H Cohen mentions he has been routinely using flavoring syrups in mineral water since at least June 7, 1808 in Philadelphia, *(July 2, 1810 – "Baltimore Whig" newspaper front page advertisement, see Appendix B).*

A few scattered bottlers would not have been enough. No, it took a series of individuals with great talents in close proximity to each other to ignite and build upon one another, plumber, druggist, marketer, chemist, glass manufacturer, etc.

Then the broader cultural change begins, a process of improvement spreads the change, and we arrive at the cultural present. Of course other products from the early period of US history, such as ice cream, have played a significant role in expanding our sugar based diet. Ice cream parlors were as widespread as soda fountains according to historical records (directories and newspapers). Ultimately mineral water was combined with ice cream in the form of floats and other concoctions.

As in life, two sides must be considered. So it is here, where the negative effects on our culture are balanced by the many positive. These include the vast soda pop industry created from these origins (mineral water pioneers). The welcome employment opportunities and widespread nurturing effect on so many associated industries such as advertising. Secondary effects where the employed are now able to help the less fortunate. It raises "*historical interaction*" questions for our future such as; will the positive and negative effects on our culture be reconciled?

The trail to the tale is so much more than just an artifact. So in conclusion, we must repeat how this book began.

An artifact is never the end of a story but the beginning of wonderful journey of adventure and discovery.

SUPPLEMENT

APPENDIX A

Mineral Water and Brewing Related U.S. Patents and Patentees
1790 – 1829

This list was compiled from some of the annual printed lists of patents which had been issued. The Patent Office records concerning these patents were destroyed in the 1836 fire. Most were not reconstructed, and the full patents are not available in the Patent Office records. These are the infamous "X" patents. Prior to 1836 patents were not issued with identifying numbers as later became the custom and practice of the U.S. Patent Office. This list may be incomplete.

Patent Date	Full Name	Patent Description	City	State
9/7/1809	HAWKINS, JOSEPH	MODE OF IMITATING NATURAL MINERAL WATERS	BALTIMORE	MD
8/16/1810	SIMONS, CHARLES D. ET AL	MODE OF SATURATING LIQUIDS WITH CARBONIC ACID GAS	CHARLESTON	SC
8/16/1810	RIONDEL, JEAN J. ET AL	MODE OF SATURATING LIQUIDS WITH CARBONIC ACID GAS	CHARLESTON	SC
6/13/1815	BEZEAU, WILLIAM	BREWING SPRUCE BEER	PHILADELPHIA	PA
12/5/1815	MARSHALL, BENJAMIN	MANUFACTURING MINERAL WATERS	ALBANY	NY
2/10/1817	EWING, JAMES S.	MAKING MINERAL WATERS	PHILADELPHIA	PA
5/4/1818	CULLEN, JOHN	MEDICATED LIQUID MAGNESIA	PHILADELPHIA	PA
4/23/1819	FAHNESTOCK, SAMUEL	APPARATUS FOR MAKING MINERAL WATERS	LANCASTER	PA
7/28/1819	HEATON, JAMES	CARBONATED MEAD	NEW YORK	NY
2/17/1820	WILLIAMS, JOHN	SPRUCE BEER	CAMBRIDGE	MA
4/5/1823	HAWKINS, JOSEPH	GIVING TEMPERATAURE TO ARTIFICIAL MINERAL WATERS	PHILADELPHIA	PA
12/19/1823	EWING, JAMES	CONSTRUCTION OF HYDRANTS	PHILADELPHIA	PA
7/19/1824	SCHIEFFELIN, JOHN L.	CARBONATED SARSASPARILLA MEAD	NEW YORK	NY
12/23/1824	LANING, JOSEPH H.	GENERATING AND CHARGING LIQUIDS WITH GAS	DAVIDSON CO	TN
5/6/1825	SEALY, RICHARD	BEER AND CIDER PUMPS	NEW YORK	NY
10/11/1828	PITKINS, LEVI	PUMP FOR DRAWING BEER, CIDER, ETC	ROCHESTER	NY

To see how the patent office fire and resulting mess of 1836/37 touched off a massive flurry of so called "***new patent***" activity throughout the US - consider just one community and one industry.

In Philadelphia a second generation of Philadelphia mineral water manufacturers and bottlers, re-patented many of the earlier patents of Ewing, Hawkins, Dyott, Cullen, etc. These earlier patents had disappeared without a trace due to the patent office fire of 1836. The patent office could do nothing about it unless the original patent holder re-constructed the patent. If re-constructed, the patent officials could deny a claim as having already been invented. But so few were re-constructed that officials could do little to deny false claims in the late 1830's and early 1840's.

Many of this second generation of mineral water related businesses can easily be identified today because they continued using the words "***Patent***" and "***Patent Improved***" on their light weight soda bottles to identify their individual mineral water and manufacturing processes, (i.e. "*double pressure*" etc.). Of course many of these patents may have been "*new inventions or improvements*" but because of the timing (right after the fire), all are painted with the same suspicions.

These bottles are all of the light weight type and nearly all were produced by the "*open / scar pontil*" manufacturing process of the late 1830's and early 1840's, (before the "*improved pontil*" process came into general use in glasshouses in the mid 1840's).

Some of the Philadelphia mineral water manufacturers and bottlers enrolled in this class of dubious "***Patent***" holders are: ***William Heiss Jr., Eugene Roussel, David Bentley, John Diehl, R. Flanagan, Peter Hall, Dr. Hartley, C.Jones, etc.*** We know this list is accurate because each left artifacts plainly embossed in the glass "***Patent***" and "***Patent Improved***", with their names embossed as well. The soda water industry was strong without all this patent activity and was growing fast because of the earlier manufacturing improvements. So these merchants would likely have done just as well without getting involved in the patent mess. Their own marketing skills would have prevailed regardless.

This flurry of patent activity was short lived however and was generally discontinued after 1844. Although a few examples pop up later, mostly related to glass manufacturing patents or bottle closure design patents, these were clearly new ideas and far outside the range of years to be considered part the infamous class of dubious inventors of the late 1830's.

This example was from just one narrow industry, in one American city – multiply this activity across America in all business fields and you can see the problem with patents from the late 1830's. Although the US patent office was rebuilt and resumed operations - numbering each patent granted, it was meaningless because they had no way to verify the truth of the claims of the applicants. Not until 15 years had passed did some semblance of truth again attach to a US patent.

APPENDIX B

The Origin of our Modern Soda Water Industry

1. Early Patents issued in the name of Joseph Hawkins

If this is the same person who was issued all the patents listed below, it is interesting to note they were issued in 3 different cities. It is interesting that during the time (1807 through 1812) he is claimed to have been in business in Philadelphia (by many historical researchers) – his patents were issued in Baltimore and New York. This confirms early city directories from Philadelphia which fail to list Joseph Hawkins or any business partnership with his name in them. However it is still possible, some Philadelphia businesses may have used Hawkins patents as was normal and accepted business practice - giving credit as legally required by any business using someone else's patent. Alternatively, Hawkins may simply have taken credit for Abraham H. Cohen's artificial mineral water manufacturing process and fountain, although I believe this is unlikely.

From patent index records, it would appear on the surface that Hawkins continued for some period of time trying to gain patents related to artificial mineral water. He appears to be using steam heat to improve the dissolving of minerals or other chemicals. This was a commonly known brewing and chemical process at that time. **It may be, that by characterizing his last patent as relating to mineral water processes he could obtain patent(s) for commonly known technology, which would have been denied otherwise.** However by 1823 many other patent holders had found other methods. Businesses no longer needed his patents. Also, many people were making specialized valves and pumps to handle water based pressurized liquids (*James S. Ewing 1817*). These methods likely formed the core methods used in the newly emerging mineral water / soda fountain businesses pioneered by early druggists and doctors in Philadelphia. Early Philadelphia engineers (plumbers) and doctors / pharmacists improved the process sufficiently so light bodied bottles could be loaded at a uniform pressure. Real sustainable business was now possible. Hawkins last patent failed to be other than a more costly curiosity already used in the brewing business and Hawkins could not claim a brewing patent for knowledge passed down for thousands of years. So his 1823 patent was useless.

Patent Date	Joseph Hawkins's Patent Descriptions	City	State
9/7/1809	MODE OF IMITATING NATURAL MINERAL WATERS	BALTIMORE	MD
4/21/1810	LAMPS AND LIQUID TO BE BURNED THEREIN	BALTIMORE	MD
6/14/1816	GENERATING STEAM	NEW YORK	NY
4/5/1823	GIVING TEMPERATAURE TO ARTIFICIAL MINERAL WATERS	PHILADELPHIA	PA

Joseph Hawkins's placed an extensive 1st advertisement on July 17, 1810 in the "*Baltimore Whig*" newspaper (see next page.). The ad ran through July 25, 1810. It mentions mineral water is sold in three bottle sizes – ½ pint, pint, & quart. All were likely heavy bodied, black glass, bottles since light bodied mineral water bottles are not found in the US or England in archaeological layers before 1825 (except for the "Cullen Egg Bottle", found herein). **Most importantly however, Hawkins describes the nature of his United States patent, as follows:**

> ***"....As the subscriber was the first that introduced the Mineral Fountains either in Europe or America, [For which he has obtained a patent from the government of the U States] and having applied a considerable portion of his life to their invention and improvement, ...".***
>
> ***(Joseph Hawkins - July 17-25, 1810)***

The significance is that Joseph Hawkins 1809 patent was for a mineral water fountain improvement or invention – not for mineral water. **Thus, John Cullen was the first to obtain a US patent for an "artificial mineral water" (soda water), whether or not many others prior to him were making artificial mineral water or not. They simply failed to obtain a patent.** The sad part of the story is that John Cullen never realized what he had and thus never capitalized on his soda water patent.

Joseph Hawkins may justly, lay claim, to being the father of America's Soda Fountain because he obtained the first American patent for a soda fountain improvement or invention. Regardless of whether many others in Europe and America were using soda fountains before 1809 is irrelevant because they did not obtain an American patent. It is unlikely Joseph Hawkins's patent was for the actual invention of a soda fountain but more likely some improvement. Remember, the patent office was required to research whether a claimed invention was common knowledge or previously invented.

The US Patent office would surely have read published articles such as found in the "*Philadelphia Medical Museum*" of 1809, pages 161–165, (an annual medical publication, 1806-1811). **Dr. Richard Green publicly describes, a method of preparing artificial Cheltenham soda water highly impregnated with carbonic acid. The President of the Royal Medical Society of Edinburgh expresses the observation at the end of the article that he doubts it is an original idea.** (In 1810, in Charleston, South Carolina, an improvement was made to this process and patented in the US – see patent chart in Appendix A – see "SIMONS & RIONDEL 8/16/1810")

Lastly, our character, John Cullen, in his 1818 advertisements, specifically mentions his soda water is available at his drugstore "Fount" or by the bottle. By 1818, soda fountains were regular features in many drugstores, especially after James S. Ewing's invention in 1817 made fountain (and bottling) mineral water equipment much safer to use – minimizing the danger of explosion. Elias Durand used this safer equipment for bottling his flavored mineral waters and as a "*fount*" in fancy imported French furniture.

HAWKINS's
Mineral Water Warehouse,
No. 7, South Gay-street.

THE Subscriber respectfully informs the Public, that having completed his apparatus upon a very extensive scale for making *Artificial Mineral Waters*, he is now prepared to supply them with SELTZER, BALLSTON, and SODA WATERS, in the highest possible perfection.

It is with confidence he now solicits the support and patronage of the public, assuring them that every exertion shall be made to give satisfaction, and to render the establishment worthy of their encouragement.

These waters, it is well known, have been strongly recommended in various complaints and with the greatest advantage by the most eminent of the faculty, both in Europe and America. The invalid, tormented by Dyspepsia, or any of its distressing symptoms, is sure to find relief in this salutary beverage; and the *Bon Vivant*, who e oppressed stomach is acid by libations of Madeira, &c. over night, is effectually cured by a glass of Soda in the morning. At the most luxurious tables, Seltzer and Madeira are often mingled, and this union of Bacchus with the Naiads is not less propitious to pleasure than to health.

To many persons languishing under disease the following information will be peculiarly acceptable, though it cannot be expected, that in every case the proposed remedies should answer:

SELTZER WATER, from its pleasant taste and Medical virtues, has been long in very general use. It has been very much recommended by physicians for its antiseptic powers, consequently for its utility in many of the febrile and other diseases of large towns. It is a powerful antiscorbutic. In bilious complaints it is particularly useful, by correcting the acrimony of that fluid, and assisting the tone of the stomach and bowels, by which pain and irritation are obviated or removed. In nervous affections it is useful by invigorating the general system, exalting the spirits, and removing weakness. To the ill effects whether nervous or bilious, which take place, as the debilitating consequence of hard living, it is peculiarly adapted. It is most refreshing and salutary after excess in eating and drinking, by allaying the feverish heat and thirst generally arising therefrom.

By gently stimulating the nerves of the stomach it increases digestion, prevents flatulencies, and promotes the secretions in general, particularly that of the kidneys.

With milk, it is a very useful remedy in consumptions, causing the milk to sit easy on the stomach. In most of the stages of the catarrh, or common cold, either in the head or lungs, it may be taken with great utility. With *wine or syrup*, it affords a most wholesome and agreeable beverage.

It is one of the safest as well as most cooling drinks for persons exhausted by much speaking, heated by dancing, or when quitting hot rooms, or crowded assemblies. It may be taken in the quantity of a common beer glass at a time.

As the subscriber was the first that introduced the Mineral Fountains either in Europe or America, [*For which he has obtained a patent from the Government of the U States*] and having applied a considerable portion of his life to their invention and improvement, he trusts that those who have been benefited by his labors, will not supercede him in favour and encouragement with a generous public, but that *he* will come in for at least an equal share of public support with those, who had it not been for his labours, would not have had it in their power to establish similar manufactories. He is willing, however, to leave it to a discerning public to determine, not according to their respective rights, but the merits of their waters being well assured that he will have abundant reason to be satisfied with their decision.

A book is opened at the warehouse for subscribers. Families can be accommodated by the single bottle, or by the dozen, in half pint, pint, or quart bottles.

☞ Orders for exportation or the country, faithfully and punctually executed.

JOSEPH HAWKINS.

July 17 d4t

CHECKS

The advertisement on the left is from July 17-25, 1810 by Joseph Hawkins of Baltimore. It authoritatively illustrates Joseph Hawkins was using and building *"soda fountains"* in 1810 at a commercial level - clearly perfected beyond an experimental level.

Thus, John Matthews of New York was not the father of the American "Soda Fountain" in the late 1830's, as is mistakenly claimed by professionals and amateurs alike.

Certainly, John Matthews improved early soda fountain designs. He successfully built a large business selling these, as did many others.

The ad on the right is from July 2, 1810 by Abraham H Cohen of Philadelphia. It illustrates that Eugene Roussel was not the first to pioneer the use of flavoring syrups in mineral water around 1839, as has been widely claimed by other researchers.

Abraham H Cohen mentions he has been routinely using flavoring syrups in mineral water since June 7, 1808 in Philadelphia :

"Independent of their medical properties, they afford the luxurious [either by themselves or united with pleasant syrups & c] a truly nectarine beverage."

Patent, census, and city directory records from 1800 – 1811 support and confirm both of these ads.

Artificial Mineral Waters.

TO THE PUBLIC.

OF all the choicest blessings bestowed on man, that of health has ever been most duly appreciated. Without this, no other can be truly enjoyed, and with it most affliction may find an alleviation. Whatever, therefore, is conducive to promote and increase this blessing, hath strong claims on public patronage and support. As tending to the object, Artificial Mineral Waters [when properly prepared] have been found effectual, as well in their physical as moral tendency; affording both an agreeable and salutary beverage, which, whilst they increase or promote health, offer a pleasing substitute for the pernicious use of ardent spirits, the inclination to which (from the exhilirating effects of these Waters) is considerably lessened, is entirely removed; being found to possess all the agreeable without their enervating or intoxicating qualities.

The pursuit of this valued blessing has led many for ages past to resort to springs famed for their salubrious or restorative powers, even when exposed to every inconvenience, or when placed at the greatest distances. Happily the important discoveries of Chemistry, hath so far obviated this difficulty, and enabled art to excite nature by an exact imitation of her process adduced from analysis—thus, their beneficial properties are encreased, or those particles found injurious, lessened, or excluded at option.

It has been generally admitted that nature in the various diseases with which mankind are afflicted, has been equally bountiful in furnishing a remedy, than which none has been found more efficacious than the use of those waters; having proved successful in many cases, where all other applications had failed. Independent of their medical properties, they afford the luxurious [either by themselves or united with pleasant syrups, &c] a truly nectarine beverage.

The importance and utility of those celebrated waters, have induced the proprietor to commence and apply every exertion to perfect an establishment so beneficial in its tendency; and his perseverance has been so far successful, as to merit the approbation and support he has received in Philadelphia, as may be evinced by the following certificates with which he was favored by some of the most eminent of the faculty in that place, viz.

We, the subscribers, have carefully examined specimens of Artificial Mineral Waters, prepared by A. H. Cohen, and find them equal to any heretofore made.

Benjamin Rush,
William P. Dewees,
Thomas Parke,
J. C. Rousseau,
M. Mongez,
J. D. Le Roche,
B. Morgan.

The following was also received from a gentleman of the most respectable Chymical knowledge, who had analysed the waters:

DEAR SIR,

I return you my thanks for the different specimens of Artificial Mineral Waters you were pleased to favor me with, at the same time, cannot but congratulate the citizens of Philadelphia, on the acquisition of an establishment which affords them so salutary and agreeable a beverage. I say, salutary, as nothing has been found more efficacious than the use of those waters in many cases, where all other applications have failed; this effect chiefly resident in a principle which I have found to exist in a considerable proportion in the waters as prepared by you; having discovered by analysing and comparing them with the natural waters, that they exceed by 3½ times the quantity of fixed air any natural aracarbonic waters ever yet discovered, whilst their other qualities are the same.—Wishing you every success so useful an establishment merits I am,

J. STUART.

Mr. A. H. Cohen.
June 7, 1808.

From the known liberality and public spirit of the citizens of Baltimore, the subscriber has been induced to extend a branch of his establishment to this city—having employed an agent for that purpose, whom he can with confidence recommend as fully competent to the correct mode of preparing these waters, having practised with him since the commencement of the establishment in this country. The proprietor is persuaded his wishes and endeavors will be zealously seconded, in the most strenuous exertions to merit and obtain public approbation.

It is expected the Waters will be ready for delivery by the 27th instant, of which due notice will be given.

A. H COHEN,
21, Water-street.

June 25 d6t

Both ads are from the "Baltimore Whig" newspaper in July 1810

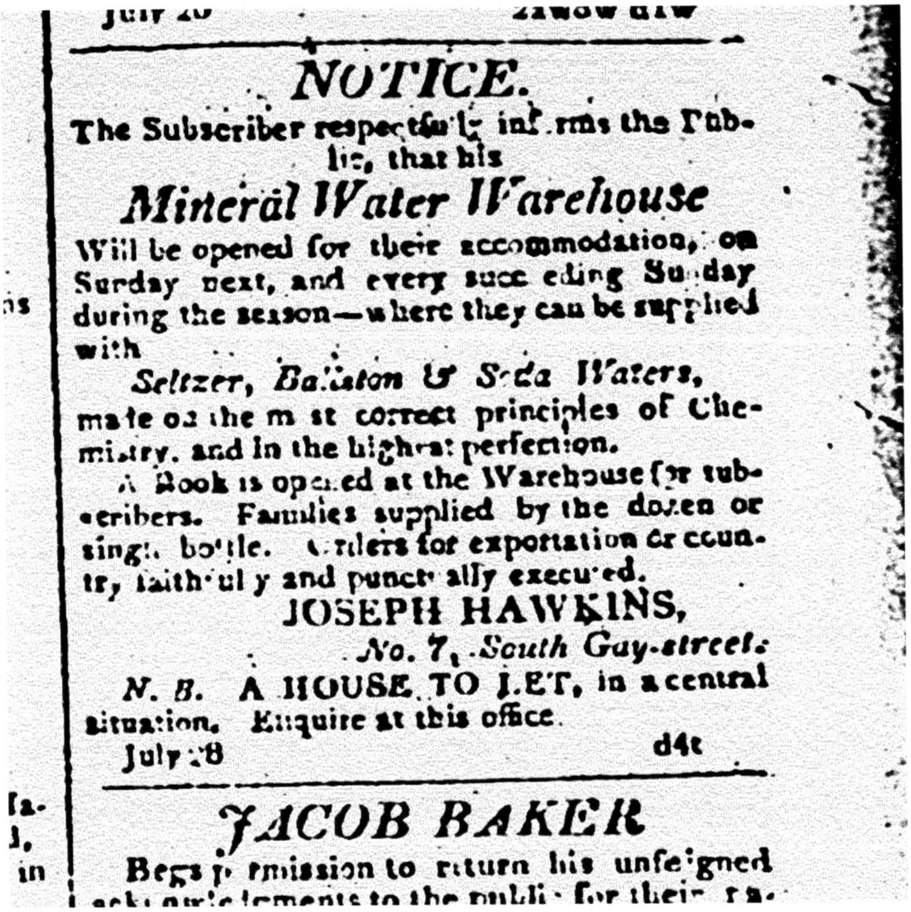

NOTICE.

The Subscriber respectfully informs the Public, that his

Mineral Water Warehouse

Will be opened for their accommodation, on Sunday next, and every succeeding Sunday during the season—where they can be supplied with

Seltzer, Ballston & Soda Waters,

made on the most correct principles of Chemistry, and in the highest perfection.

A Book is opened at the Warehouse for subscribers. Families supplied by the dozen or single bottle. Orders for exportation or country, faithfully and punctually executed.

JOSEPH HAWKINS,

No. 7, South Gay-street.

N. B. A HOUSE TO LET, in a central situation. Enquire at this office.

July 28 d4t

JACOB BAKER

Begs permission to return his unfeigned

Above, is Joseph Hawkins's 2nd advertisement in the "*Baltimore Whig*" newspaper on August 6, 1810. It shows he was operating a mineral water warehouse at No. 7 South Gay Street and selling his product by the bottle – there is no mention of a United States patent.

John Matthews, G.S.Twitchell, and many others, built their businesses by a process of continuous improvement, basing their original soda water and equipment businesses on the expired patents of James S. Ewing, Joseph Hawkins's, John Cullen, and others.

Most biographical reference books overlook this historical context and tend to relate sensational antidotes and obvious fictional stories with no real foundation. These stories are then reference quoted over and over until they are believed by the academic and lay communities. John Matthew's biographical material is a good example of overblown claims and fictional accounts of manufacturing methods that likely never occurred.

Eugene Roussel is another example - often mistakenly credited with pioneering the use of flavoring syrups in mineral waters, when in fact he merely copied their use from others. Professionals and amateurs alike have greatly exaggerated his role based on poorly researched biographical material, and reference quoted over and over again.

2. Early Patents issued in the name of James Ewing

The primary reason Joseph Hawkins and other early pioneers failed to establish the US artificial mineral water industry is because the fountain and manufacturing equipment they used was terribly unstable (until mid 1817). **Although Hawkins, Hamilton, Schweppe, Cohen, Shaw, Silliman, Physick, Seaman, and so many others claimed to have devoted significant resources and time to the invention and improvement of mineral water manufacturing equipment - their equipment had a reputation of exploding.** Also, this early equipment required constant maintenance because of internal corrosion. It was largely incapable of filling a container to a consistent pressure or to maintain consistent pressure inside the various mixing tanks. It was therefore even more dangerous if heat was used in the process. The most common early use was as a fountain which allowed for immediate distribution of product to the waiting customers, greatly reducing the risk of explosion because of the constant reduction of pressure.

In 1817 James S. Ewing became the unsung hero of the artificial mineral water industry. His invention spread from Philadelphia outward, across regions and continents. The right combination of individuals with complementary skills existed within a few blocks of Ewing. This combination lead to soda water bottling on a large scale, in bottles, that were much lighter in weight than the black glass "*cannon balls*" previously used. T.W. Dyott advertised many thousands of these lighter mineral water bottles on hand by the early 1820's. This transition also started to occur in England as well for the same reason as it did in the US and allowed Schweppe & Co to slowly switchover from stoneware bottles to glass bottles. The archaeological record supports this theory because no glass bottles, as described in the patents and advertisements have been found before the mid 1820's artifact layers, (either in England or the United States (except for Cullen's Egg Bottle)). That raises the question, is there any historical evidence supporting the lack of an archaeological record?

The answer is yes! October 22, 1818, James S. Ewing describes a "*Patent Improved Hydrant*", (water hydrant), in a newspaper ad, for which he has obtained a US patent. The only patent which James S. Ewing had obtained at that time is described in *US Patent Office* index records as, "*Making Mineral Waters*" granted on February 10, 1817. The "*Hydrant*" invention is clearly used for controlling liquids under pressure. So is there any evidence this was used in mineral water manufacturing equipment? Yes!

December 14, 1825, H & J Ewing & Co, again advertise their, "*Patent Improved Hydrant*", (water hydrant), as well as, valves, pumps, and other products they manufacture and sell. (James S. Ewing had passed away and the family continued with the manufacturing business). In this advertisement, near the bottom of a long column with a woodcut graphic picture of their hydrant, H & J Ewing & Co. states:

> ***"...Their Mineral Water Apparatus is superior to any other in use. It effectively guards the operator from danger of explosion, and the water cannot come in contact with brass or copper in any part...."***

May 7 dtf

PATENT IMPROVED HYDRANT.

THE subscriber has constructed a Hydrant calculated to obviate the most important defects of those in common use. To prevent freezing in winter, the waste water is discharged instantly after drawing. The cock will last many years, whereas those in common use are seldom tight after 12 or 18 months, when they begin to leak into the ground and subject the owner to a fine of five dollars. The most probable repair that may be required, can be done on the spot; but if it requires to be taken up, it can be done without removing the pavement, thus avoiding the expense of digging and repaving, and the inconvenience of having the yard broken. During the time of repairing, the supply of water will not be interrupted, this being provided for in the construction of the Hydrants. Those who are desirous of viewing this improvement, are requested to call on the subscriber, at No. 231, Chesnut street, near Eighth.

A fresh importation of WATER CLOUTS of every description.

JAMES S. EWING.

October 9 fwtu6w

A PARTNER WANTED.

WHO can advance from 7 to 10,000 dollars in the wholesale grocery buisiness, at an old established stand. A line addressed to H. R. T. through the medium of the Post Office, will be at

James S Ewing's advertisement for his remote controlled, no leak, freeze proof - safety pressure valves (the key parts of his patent improved hydrant invention and mineral water bottling and manufacturing equipment).

This newspaper image appeared October 22, 1818 in the, "*Aurora General Advertiser*" of Philadelphia, Pennsylvania (page 4 column 3). **It mentions his remote safety hydrant valve is patented.**

The only patent James S. Ewing had in 1818 was described by US Patent Office index records as, "*Making Mineral Waters*" granted on February 10, 1817.

Courtesy of "*The Library Company of Philadelphia*"
(Call number 4-B-3-5)

reduced prices, and on liberal terms. oct 10—d

PATENT IMPROVED HYDRANT.

Recommended by the City Councils and the Watering Committee, honoured with the Scott Premium, by the Agricultural Society, and with the Extra Magellanic Premium by the American Philosophical Society.

The Lever Hydrant, which has lately received the Extra Magellanic Premium of the American Philosophical Society, has been used throughout Philadelphia, and proved an effectual safeguard against freezing, even in the coldest winters.

It cannot be left leaking through carelessness.

It will probably last more than 20 years.

Its cocks will last longer than any other part of the Hydrant, but common cocks wear out and leak in one year.

It is the cheapest and best Hydrant now in use.

All repairs will be insured for one dollar.

It can be taken up for repairing, without digging or breaking the pavement.

Common Hydrants at very low prices.

Second hand ones nearly as good as new, from one to two dollars each.

Hydrants of all kinds repaired.

Pumps for country houses, which will raise water from any distance or depth, distribute it through the rooms for baths or for safety, and project it 40 feet over the roof.

Having engaged a constant supply of Iron Pipes, to be put up in alleys where water is to be distributed to several houses, the subscribers will lay them on the most reasonable terms.

They also make Lead Pumps, Bath and Water Closets, and do all kinds of Lead Work.

Their Mineral Water Apparatus is superior to any other in use. It effectually guards the operator from danger of explosion, and the water cannot come in contact with brass or copper in any part.

Turning of any description in metals, executed with neatness and dispatch.

IMPROVED PATENT HYDRANTS.

The Subscribers having obtained a Patent for the above improvement, caution all persons from making, selling, or using them without their consent.

H. & J. EWING & Co.

Plumbers, Lodge street, back of No. 231, Chesnut street. nov 8—dtfcp1t

Cough Drops or Indian Specific.

This newspaper ad with woodcut image, appeared December 14, 1825 in, *"The Union, United States Gazette and True American"* of Philadelphia, Pennsylvania (page 4 column 1).

It mentions the American Philosophical Society's ***"Extra Magellanic Premium"*** award given to Ewing (in 1823) for his remote controlled pressure valve used in hydrants *(US Patent - 12/19/1823),* and mineral water equipment *(US Patent – 2/10/1817)*, etc.

Near the bottom, Ewing & Co. describe their "explosion proof" mineral water manufacturing equipment as being superior to any other in use. This is what allowed bottling on a commercial scale and began the modern soda industry we see today.

This bottling equipment was widely copied in the US and Europe.

Courtesy of "*The Library Company of Philadelphia*"

James S. Ewing and his family list their business address as Chestnut Street from 1813 until 1825 - within a few blocks of John Cullen, T.W. Dyott, and Elias Durand. John Cullen moves to Virginia, James S. Ewing passes away, Elias Durand looking for opportunity, moves from Baltimore to Philadelphia to take over the mineral water fountain and druggist business of the Ewing family since James had passed away.

However, the Ewing family did not sell all parts of their business - they retained their manufacturing business for hydrants, valves, pumps, and mineral water equipment - as their December 14, 1825 advertisement states. Durand's newly purchased druggist business, soda fountain business, and mineral water bottling business (using the new lighter bodied bottles), is successful and soon Durand has many other competitors using Ewing's equipment to manufacture mineral waters.

What made all this possible was that the finest mineral water manufacturing equipment in the world was available right on *Chestnut Street* and soon everyone copied it. Of course by the late 1830's, Ewing's patents had expired and also were revoked by Congress due to the 1836 patent office fire which destroyed all the patent records. Using this legal void, other American based competitors soon took advantage of the situation - such as John M. Matthews of NYC, Eugene Roussel, of Philadelphia, William Heiss Jr. of Philadelphia, and English competitors such as Schweppe & Co -, quickly copying Ewing's MW equipment and the soda water bottling and soda fountain industry grew and spread rapidly.

We recognize the evolution of Ewing's invention even today. The modern freeze valve used in our homes to protect our pipes in winter from freezing, the hydrants in our public water systems, the common lever beer tap used in so many bars and restaurants around the world, remote controlled valves in many thousands of bottling plants around the world – hydraulic valves around the world and now in space - all can trace their origins to Ewing's *Patent Water Hydrant's.* Everyone owes an immeasurable debt of gratitude to him.

This is one of America's greatest inventions due to its broad influence over the centuries and around the globe - and yet is unknown and unrecognized. James S. Ewing, was awarded one of America's most prestigious prizes for his lever hydrant invention. The *American Philosophical Society* awarded their "*Magellanic Premium Award*" to him in 1823. This award is still given to other great Americans and all winners can be viewed on the internet on the APS web site. The *American Philosophical Society* was founded by Benjamin Franklin in the 1700's. Lastly, James Ewing was granted a second US patent on December 19, 1823, described in the US patent index as "*Construction of Hydrants*".

Patent Date	James Ewing's Patent Descriptions	City	State
2/10/1817	MAKING MINERAL WATERS	PHILADELPHIA	PA
12/19/1823	CONSTRUCTION OF HYDRANTS	PHILADELPHIA	PA

Your author has obtained copies of James S Ewing's handwritten letter and drawings from 1823 describing his invention in detail including full background information on his motivation and historical context of the Philadelphia water system in the early US period (1800 – 1823). Wonderful details such as the actual costs to construct a cistern at that time and so much more. These actual drawings it is hoped will be used to reconstruct Ewing's second patent in cooperation with the US patent office.

All of "*Appendix B*" material will be explored in far more detail in succeeding volumes in this series and is a prerequisite to them.

Partial list of Philadelphia Directory entries for James S. Ewing & Family

Year	Listed Name	Philadelphia Address	Occupation	Ref
1810	(not listed)			49
1811	(not listed)			49
1813	Ewing, James S.	209 Chestnut St.	Apothecary & c	46
1814	Ewing, James S.	209 Chestnut St.	Apothecary & c	50
1816	Ewing, James S.	211 Chestnut St.	Apothecary & c	49
1817	Ewing, James S.	243 Chestnut St.	Apothecary & c	49
1818	Ewing, James S.	231 Chestnut St.	Apothecary & c	46
1819	Ewing, James S.	231 Chestnut St.	Druggist & Plumber	46
1820	Ewing, James S.	231 Chestnut St.	Druggist & Plumber	36
1821	Ewing, James S.	231 Chestnut St.	Druggist & Plumber	51
1822	Ewing, James S.	231 Chestnut St.	Druggist & Plumber	51
1823	Ewing, Jas.S.	231 Chestnut St.	Druggist & Plumber	2
1824	Ewing, Jas.S.	231 Chestnut St.	Druggist & Plumber	2
1825	Ewing, H.J. & Co.	231 Chestnut St.	Druggists & Plumbers	37
1828	Ewing, Jacob	306 Sassafras St.	Plumber	2
1829	Ewing, Jacob & Wm.	8 S 8th St.	Plumbers	2
1830	Ewing, Jacob & Wm.	23 S 8th St.	Plumbers	2
1835	Ewing, Jacob	21 & 23 S 8th St.	Plumber	2
1837	Ewing, Jacob	23 S 8th St.	Plumber	2
1840	Ewing, Jacob O.	23 S 8th St.	Plumber and Manuf,	1

The preceding material in *(Appendix B" - The Origin of our Modern Soda Water Industry)* is not 100% conclusive and other competing theories are possible. Your author's theory is supported by substantial OSD material cited herein, which must be overcome by conflicting OSD material of equal or greater authority and weight. My peers are invited to participate in bringing further illumination to this subject but should not expect any response to reference quoting or minor differences in opinion. Only, "*Original source documents*" should be used in this evolving research. All OSD material should be verifiable, material, and substantive - as is the OSD material your author has presented herein for your consideration.

20 Feb 1823

49

Ultra quam satis est, virtutem si petat ipsam

Cover page of James S. Ewing's Magellanic Award presentation document.

Dr Robert Patterson Senr

President of the American

Philosophical Society

read 21 Feby 1823

for Magellanic Premium

Envelope page of James S. Ewing's Magellanic Award presentation document
Courtesy of *"American Philosophical Society"*, Philadelphia

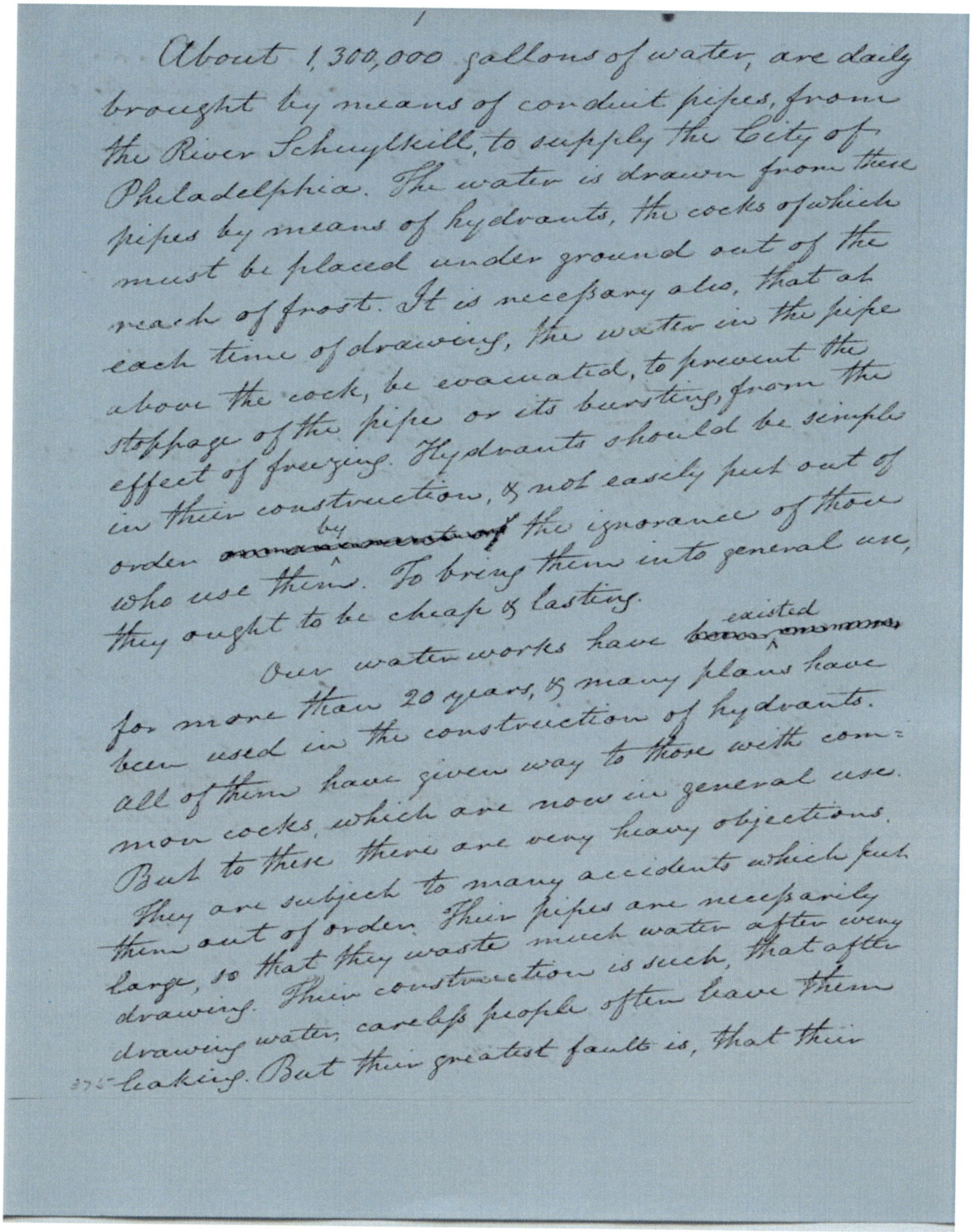

1

About 1,300,000 gallons of water, are daily brought by means of conduit pipes, from the River Schuylkill, to supply the City of Philadelphia. The water is drawn from these pipes by means of hydrants, the cocks of which must be placed under ground out of the reach of frost. It is necessary also, that at each time of drawing, the water in the pipe above the cock, be evacuated, to prevent the stoppage of the pipe or its bursting, from the effect of freezing. Hydrants should be simple in their construction, & not easily put out of order by the ignorance of those who use them. To bring them into general use, they ought to be cheap & lasting.

Our water works have existed for more than 20 years, & many plans have been used in the construction of hydrants. All of them have given way to those with common cocks, which are now in general use. But to these there are very heavy objections. They are subject to many accidents which put them out of order. Their pipes are necessarily large, so that they waste much water after every drawing. Their construction is such, that after drawing water, careless people often leave them leaking. But their greatest fault is, that their

Page 1 of James S. Ewing's Magellanic Award presentation document
Courtesy of *"American Philosophical Society"*, Philadelphia

2

cocks wear out so fast, as to cause a daily leakage
of more than $\frac{1}{3}$ of all the water brought into the City,
& an annual expense nearly equal to the water rent.
From this cause of leakage they are very subject to freezing
in winter. This great leakage has been accurately
ascertained by careful experiments, which have prov=
ed the average loss of water from them, after having
been 2 years in use, to be equal to 173 gallons each,
per day, or about 3 times as much as the supply of a
family. The quantity thus lost, would be sufficient
for the Northern Liberties & Southwark. If a strict
administration of our laws, should constrain the
owners to repair them as soon as their leakage equals
the quantity consumed in a family, the cost of repairs to
the citizens using the water, would be at least twenty
thousand dollars per annum. In the whole City of
Philada only 4000 houses are supplied with the
Schuylkill water. This scanty demand, can only arise
from the vexations of leakage from the hydrants, &
pipes, & their enormous annual expense. If these dis=
advantages can be overcome, & the water be extend
ed to the liberties, it is highly probable that the reve=
nue from the water, may be doubled by extending
its supply.

The writer believes that he has contrived a hy=
drant worked by a lever of simple construction, which will last many
years, will cost very little for repairs, & will neither
freeze nor leak, even through the carelessness of those who
use it. Though it shuts off the water 3 feet underground,
the whole content of the pipe, hitherto termed waste–

Page 2 of James S. Ewing's Magellanic Award presentation document
Courtesy of *"American Philosophical Society"*, Philadelphia

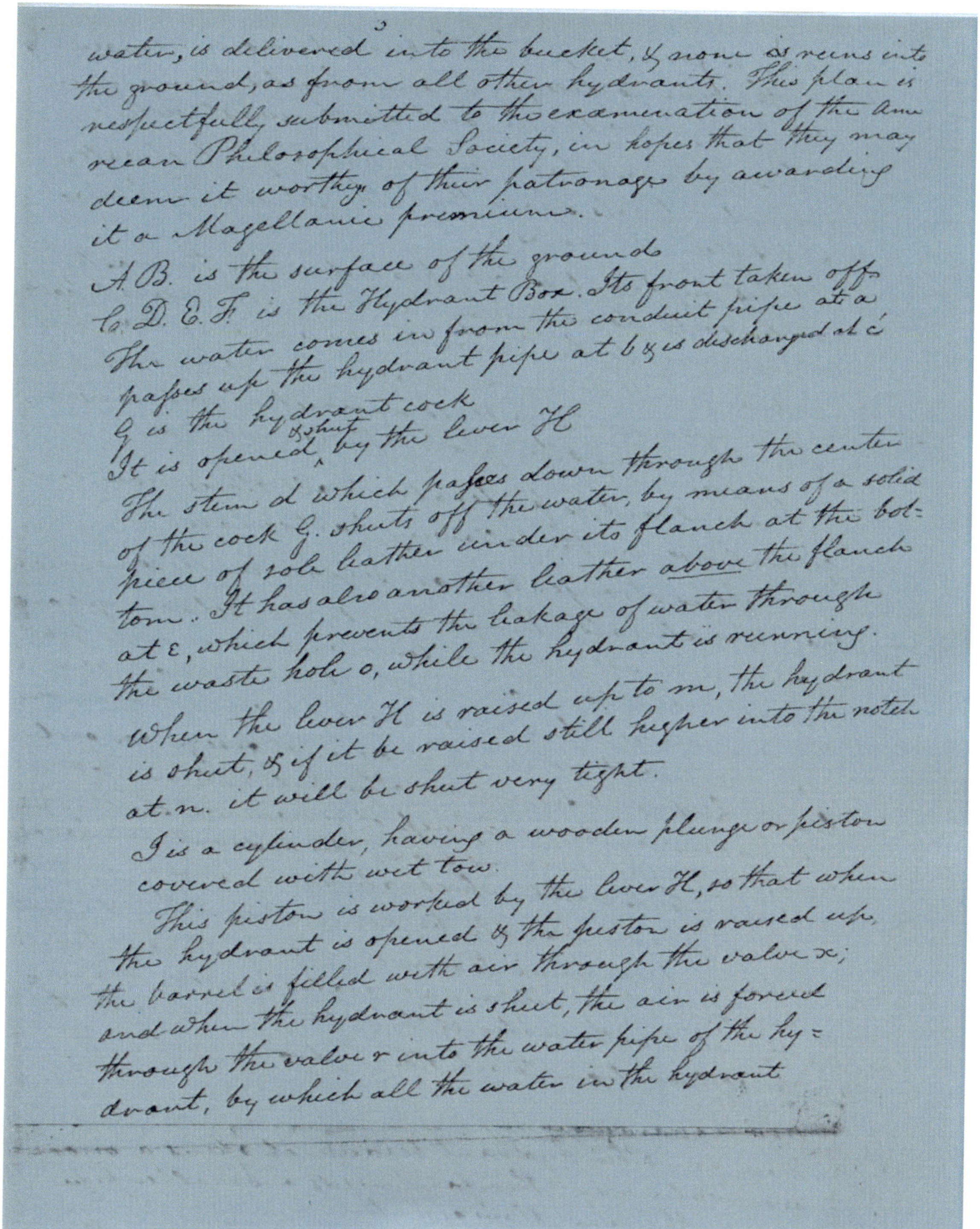
3

water, is delivered into the bucket, & none is runs into the ground, as from all other hydrants. This plan is respectfully submitted to the examination of the American Philosophical Society, in hopes that they may deem it worthy of their patronage by awarding it a Magellanic premium.

A B. is the surface of the ground
C. D. E. F. is the Hydrant Box. Its front taken off.
The water comes in from the conduit pipe at a
passes up the hydrant pipe at b & is discharged at c
G is the hydrant cock
It is opened & shut by the lever H

The stem d which passes down through the center of the cock G. shuts off the water, by means of a solid piece of sole leather under its flanch at the bottom. It has also another leather above the flanch at e, which prevents the leakage of water through the waste hole o, while the hydrant is running.

When the lever H is raised up to m, the hydrant is shut, & if it be raised still higher into the notch at n. it will be shut very tight.

I is a cylinder, having a wooden plunger or piston covered with wet tow.

This piston is worked by the lever H, so that when the hydrant is opened & the piston is raised up, the barrel is filled with air through the valve x; and when the hydrant is shut, the air is forced through the valve r into the water pipe of the hydrant, by which all the water in the hydrant

Page 3 of James S. Ewing's Magellanic Award presentation document
Courtesy of *"American Philosophical Society"*, Philadelphia

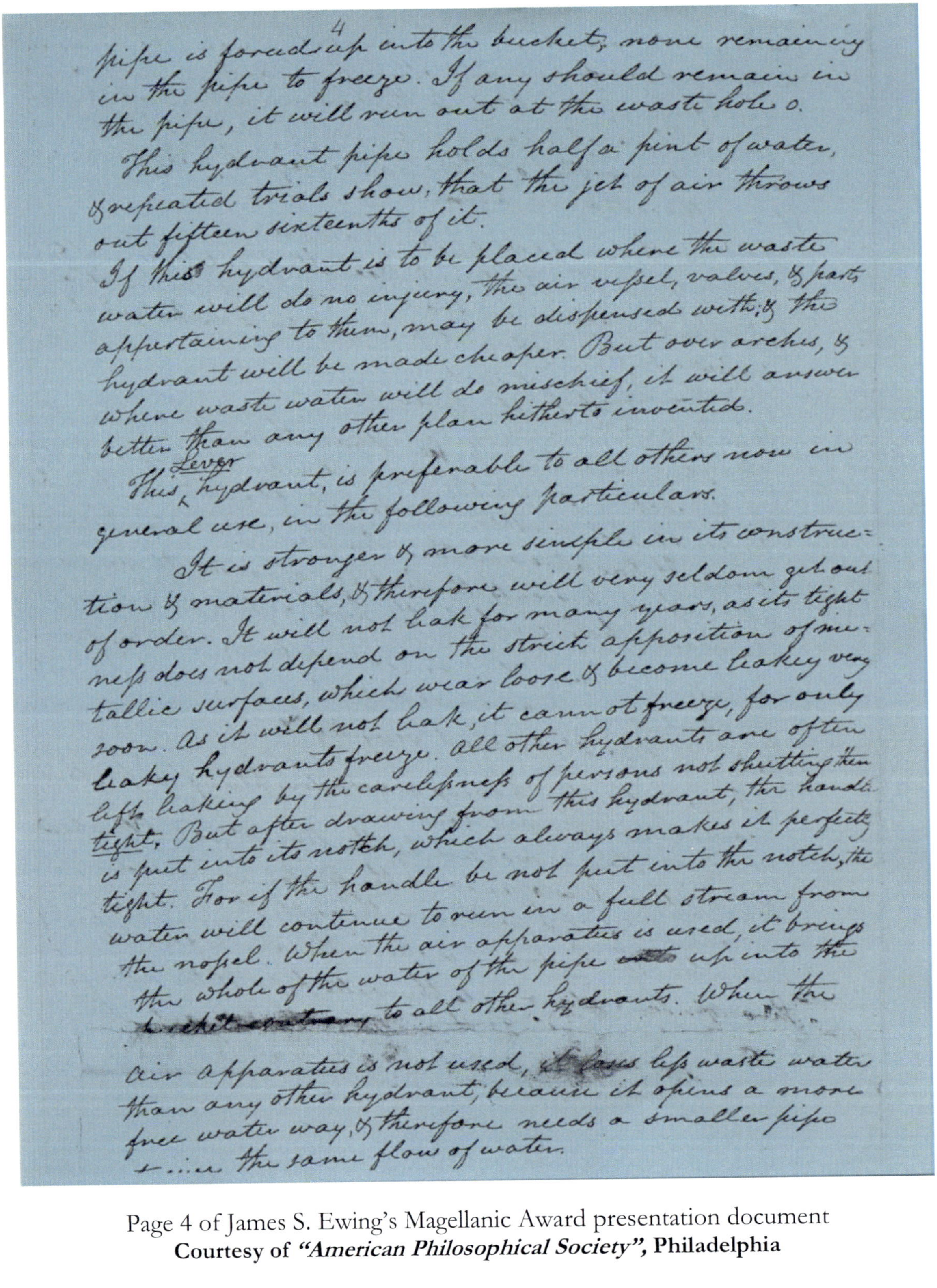
4

pipe is forced up into the bucket, none remaining in the pipe to freeze. If any should remain in the pipe, it will run out at the waste hole o.

This hydrant pipe holds half a pint of water, & repeated trials show, that the jet of air throws out fifteen sixteenths of it.

If this hydrant is to be placed where the waste water will do no injury, the air vessel, valves, & parts appertaining to them, may be dispensed with; & the hydrant will be made cheaper. But over arches, & where waste water will do mischief, it will answer better than any other plan hitherto invented.

This lever hydrant, is preferable to all others now in general use, in the following particulars.

It is stronger & more simple in its construction & materials, & therefore will very seldom get out of order. It will not leak for many years, as its tightness does not depend on the strict apposition of metallic surfaces, which wear loose & become leakey very soon. As it will not leak, it cannot freeze, for only leakey hydrants freeze. All other hydrants are often left leaking by the carelessness of persons not shutting them tight. But after drawing from this hydrant, the handle is put into its notch, which always makes it perfectly tight. For if the handle be not put into the notch, the water will continue to run in a full stream from the nossel. When the air apparatus is used, it brings the whole of the water of the pipe ~~into~~ up into the ~~bucket contrary~~ to all other hydrants. When the air apparatus is not used, ~~it loses~~ less waste water than any other hydrant, because it opens a more free water way, & therefore needs a smaller pipe [illegible] the same flow of water.

Page 4 of James S. Ewing's Magellanic Award presentation document
Courtesy of *"American Philosophical Society"*, Philadelphia

5

As this Hydrant will always be tight, will very seldom need repairs & though extended to any depth, can be taken up without digging, it will give rise to a very useful improvement in our water works that of having clear Cold-Water-hydrants, that shall answer all the purposes of Cisterns, at one fifth of their usual expense. This will be done by making the hydrants 12 or 15 feet deep, & connecting them with Reservoirs formed of materials which conduct heat at that depth, in which the water will have become clear & cold, & bringing it up through pipes which will not alter its temperature.

Cisterns cost from one hundred to two hundred dollars & are often rendered useless by cracks which let in filthy water. Besides which, many lots have no room to contain them. But the Cold-Water Hydt. can be put where there may be room for any hydt. & its reservoir may be put under the Cellar. No dirty water can penetrate this reservoir because of the internal pressure.

This plan of a cold-water-hydrant the Writer means to execute after the ground becomes free from frost, & he hopes that its being mentioned here will not be the means of its being suggested to others, who may anticipate him.

379

Page 5 of James S. Ewing's Magellanic Award presentation document
Courtesy of *"American Philosophical Society"*, Philadelphia

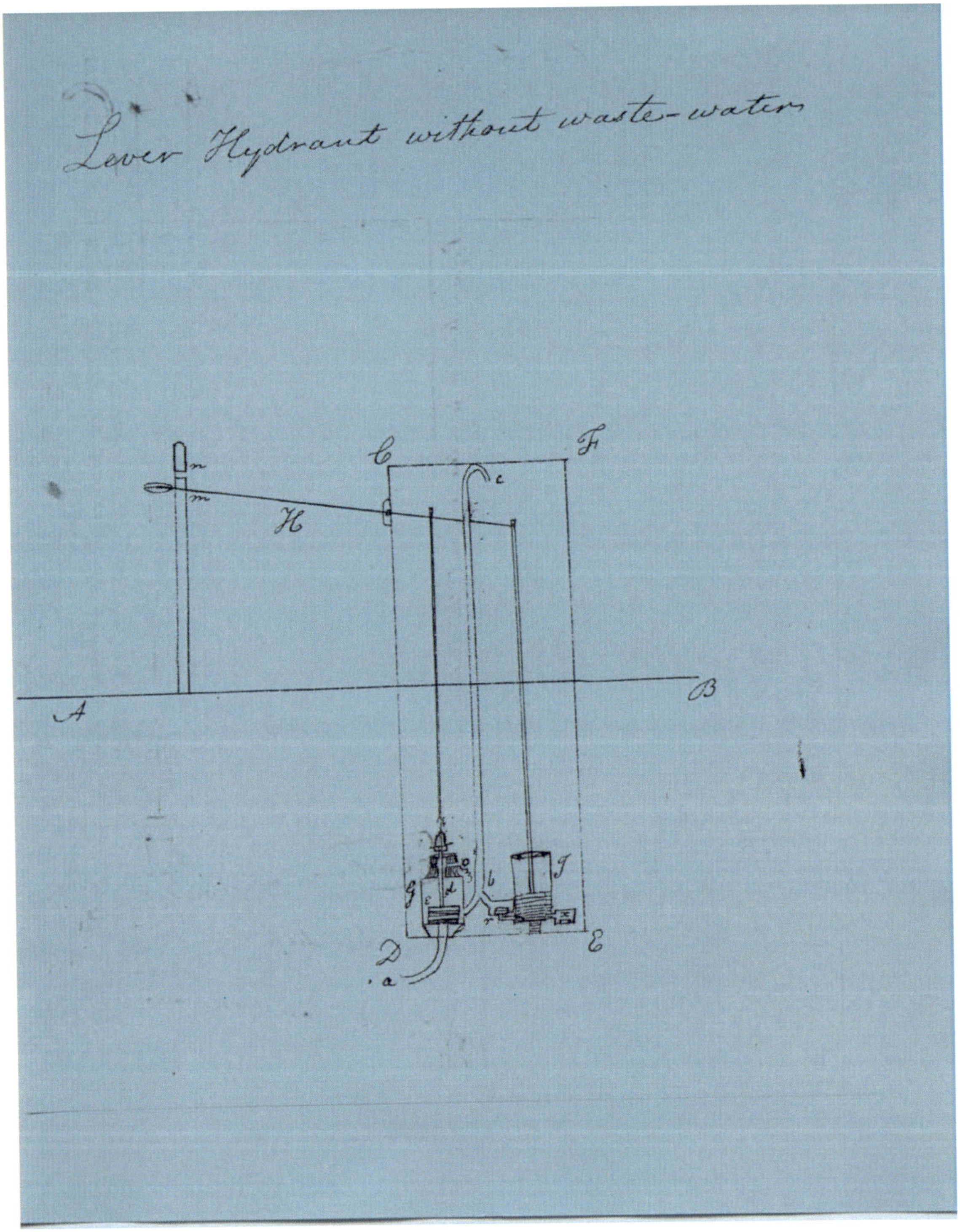

Page 6 of James S. Ewing's Magellanic Award presentation document
First type of patented valve: Remote Lever Controlled No-Leak Safety High Pressure Liquid Hydrant Valve & Assembly
(Used on Mineral Water manufacturing equipment & fountains)
Courtesy of *"American Philosophical Society"*, Philadelphia

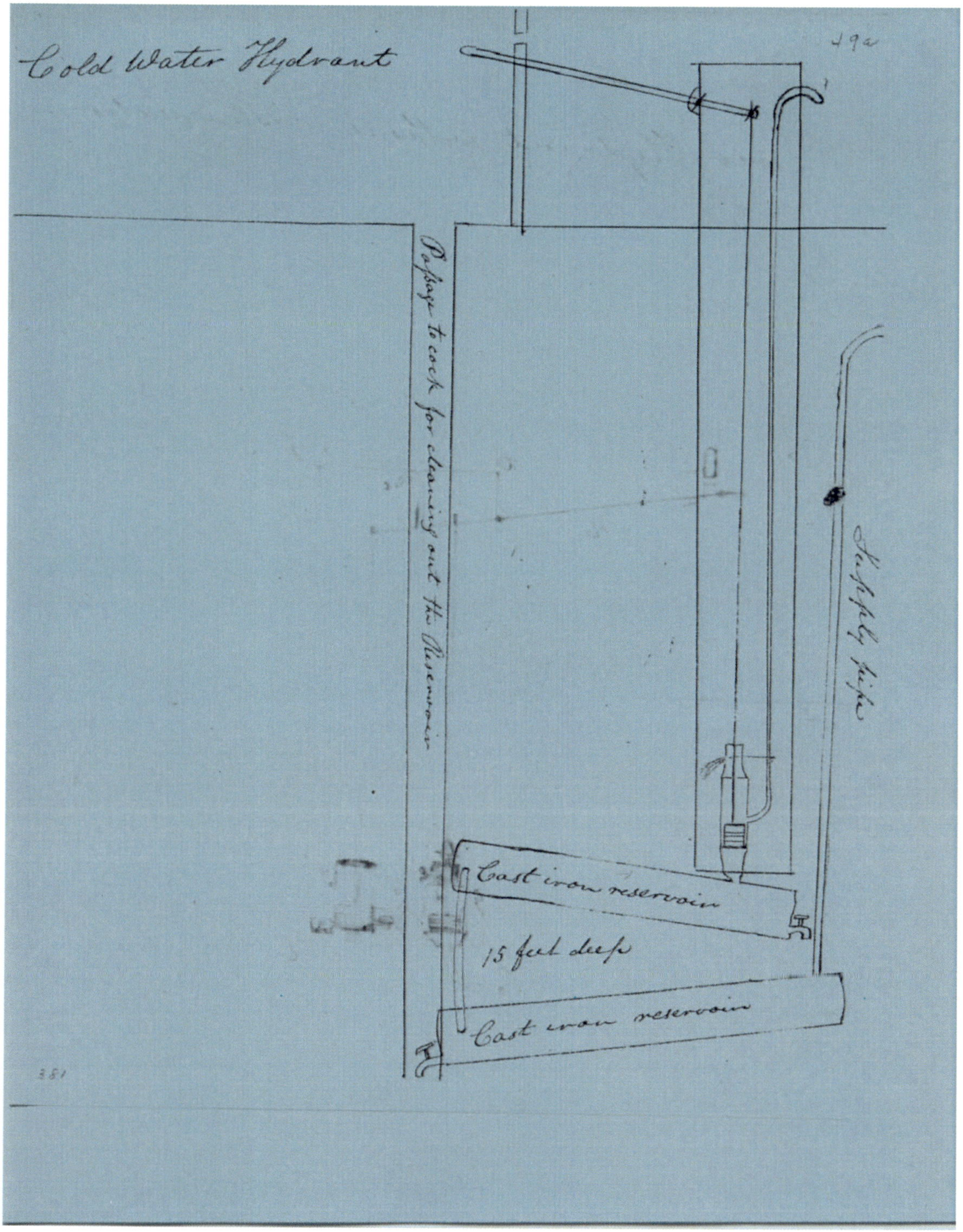

Page 7 of James S. Ewing's Magellanic Award presentation document
Second type of patented valve: Remote Lever Controlled No-Leak Safety High Pressure Liquid Hydrant Valve & Assembly with waste water (Freeze valve)
(Used on Mineral Water manufacturing equipment & fountains)
Courtesy of *"American Philosophical Society"*, Philadelphia

APPENDIX C

Summary
The Egg Bottles:

Most early (pre-1830) egg bottles are lettered vertically (parallel to the length of the bottle). The Cullen bottle however is lettered horizontally in rows around the middle of the bottle. This is somewhat unusual in egg bottles.

The first generation of egg bottles, which I believe currently includes only the Cullen bottle, have the earliest style of manufactured top, not found on any other known American or English egg bottle - the top is a sheared (sharp) lip with a 1700's style ¼' thin glass ring attached just under the cut off neck. Black glass bottles of the 1700's commonly had such a string lip design. It was continued on black glass bottles and a few decorative American flasks into the early 1800's and occasionally later. In mineral water bottles, this manufacturing method evolved into the more traditional attached tapered top, squared top, and rounded tops. The difference was the cut off neck became hidden under the attached glass ring (or top) and the neck was no longer exposed in later mineral water bottles. Perhaps the most impressive feature is the delicate light weight wall design of Cullen's egg bottle at such an early period. Only in Philadelphia was precise liquid pressure loading equipment available in 1818, which could prevent explosions in thin walled bottles. At this time I believe Cullen's egg bottle is the earliest known embossed egg bottle that is confirmed by historical records (1818), manufacturing design (1750 - 1820), and archaeological context (1815 -1820). Cullen's bottle likely preceded the known Schweppe's egg bottles of 79 Margaret Street London (1809 -1831), and the David Grant bottles of Pickett Street London (1817-1830) for the reasons as mentioned below.

The second generation of egg bottles, which includes most early (pre-1830) English egg bottles (Schweppe's 79 Margaret Street; Grant's Patent Soda Water, Pickett Street; etc.), were finished with an applied ring glass top - the earliest are narrow rings (5/16 - 3/8 in), later they are larger and more closely resemble the blob or taper tops used through the remainder of the 19th century. These both have flat bases. No double collars are known on these early eggs. It is not likely English egg bottles were used before the early 1820's because of the danger of explosion as discussed in the next section.

Although it is possible a few of the Schweppe's 79 Margaret Street egg bottles preceded the Cullen egg bottle, it is not likely based on the known evidence which includes; manufacturing methods, historical records, archaeological context, and artifacts to date. There is no known archaeological context indicating an earlier date, that I could locate, for any Schweppes egg bottles having the 79 Margaret Street address. Also, the Guildhall museum (*Museum of London*) archaeological context records were either missing, or do not exist for the known David Grant, Pickett Street, egg bottle dug by Ivor Noel Hume before his American assignments in a cesspool pit behind the museum. The Grant bottle has a flat base with pontil and narrow attached ring top similar to the early Schweppe's egg bottles.

The earliest English historical records, with direct dated evidence mentioning egg bottles at a commercial level are Schweppe's invoices offering glass egg bottles as an option to their normal stoneware bottles and dated 1821. This is confirmed by noted English researcher Olive Talbot in her extensive work titled *"The Evolution of Glass Bottles for Carbonated Drinks"*, published in *"Post Medieval Archaeology" Vol. 8, 1974; Page 39.*

There are two egg shaped stoneware bottles in the possession of Cadbury Schweppes (*currently a division of Pepsico, Inc.*) in brown salt glaze exterior finish and both have the 79 Margaret Street address on them. These were the actual Schweppe mineral water bottles from 1792 – 1820. If any glass egg bottles were used prior to 1820, it was likely experimental only.

The manufacturing methods used in making the known Schweppes bottles of 79 Margaret Street and Grant bottles of Pickett Street, were generally not used on light weight glass bottles until the mid 1820's (attached ring tops) and small flat bases. The earlier glass bottle manufacturing style for light weight bottles, (prior to 1820), was a sheared lip with a string glass lip ring and rounded open pontilled base. The later manufacturing processes of the 1820's and early 1830's used flat bases as seen on the known Schweppes examples of 79 Margaret Street - so as to facilitate a speedier manufacturing process in making egg bottles (*this allowed for an easier and stronger pontil process*). It was not until the pontil process was eliminated that round or pointed bottoms returned (as seen in the Schweppes bottles of 51 Berners Street (1831-1895).

The third generation of egg bottles, from 1830 – 1835, were transitional between pontils and non-pontils. They were often made of dark olive or black glass. (see London's Paul & Harfield/5 Bow Street/Covent Garden (1833), New York's Aspinwall & Rushton 81 William & 110 Broadway (1833-1835), New York's G.D.Coggeshall 421 Pearl Street (1829-1833), *inter alia*). These had small flat bases similar to the Schweppes. Many were sand pontilled instead of open pontilled.

The fourth generation of egg bottles in 1835 - 1855 were normally not pontilled (see Merchant's Soda Water, Lockport N.Y (1845); Schweppes 51 Berners & Oxford Street London (1831-1895); Chapman Soda, Baltimore Maryland (1835-1845); *inter alia*). A pontilled example would be A.T.Blake, Cincinnati Ohio (1838 - 1841). A few retained the small flat base design even though not pontilled. Examples are Chapman of Baltimore and early Schweppes 51 Berners Street bottles. These evolved into "ten pin" egg designs such as Jones Patent Mineral Water and Shock & Jones from Philadelphia. Some areas such as Baltimore developed their own unique style of egg bottle in a rich tapestry of colors.

The earliest Schweppes 51 Berners Street bottles are nearly identical to the known 79 Margaret Street bottles, in color (olive green), weight of glass, embossing style, font size, lip finish, and capacity. They probably date close to each other (1825 –1835). The only difference being that one is pontilled and one is not.

Fourth generation egg bottles were not limited to the US and England. Many other countries have wonderful egg bottle examples of their own, (i.e. Canada). Some of the earliest patent holders involved with bottling artificial mineral water are from France, Switzerland, Canada (Quebec City), and Germany. There are others as well.

Many different styles of egg bottles (sometimes called torpedo) followed in the period after 1855. They can be found in such faraway places as India, Hong Kong, Australia, and New Zealand.

Summary
The Mineral Water Manufacturing / Fountain Equipment:

The bottling equipment pictured in early English / Irish patents shows a tapered shaft spigot control valve used for filling of mineral water containers. This type of brass valve was leaky under pressure and could not handle high pressure that often built up and would then explode unexpectedly.

Often the valve control shaft would separate from the tapered body even after relatively minor use and shoot out like a bullet. The brass end pin or screw would deform under pressure and could no longer hold the valve together. Equally dangerous was the fact that these valves could not fill containers to a consistent or repeatable pressure. They allowed much higher pressures in glass containers than could be safely handled – the result - explosion of the bottle causing death or serious injury - even if the equipment itself did not explode.

Thus, if light weight glass bottles were used, a serious risk of injury existed for the operator because they would often explode in their face. I found **no** remote controlled valves pictured in any of the European patent drawings that I examined (mentioned below).

American patent drawings were burned in the great fire of 1836 at the US patent office in Washington D.C. However I was able to locate the 1823 drawings of James S. Ewing and was able to reconstruct his patents of 1817 and 1823 which clearly show the many safety features and remote control valves necessary to prevent explosions. Ewing's advertisements of 1825 claim, a superiority to prevent explosions, over all other known mineral water equipment marketed at that time.

Even in grocery stores in the 1970's, glass soda bottles routinely exploded on store shelves for no apparent reason. Plastic bottles largely ended the danger in the 1980's.

Before 1820, these frequent accidents with mineral water manufacturing equipment (and fountain equipment) resulted in many deaths and serious injuries. Taper shaft, soft metal, liquid control valves were manufactured from the late 1700's up through and into the early 1850's. Several pictures follow of a two archaeologically recovered tapered spigot valves from 1830's as confirmed by artifact context and historic record (*based on the embossed manufacturer's name stamped in the metal*).

In America this situation was partially avoided by the commercial development of the soda fountain in the 1800 through 1810 period (Joseph Hawkins, Sillman, Physick, etc.) The soda fountain allowed for the steady and continual reduction of pressure due to the waiting customers to be served. Bottling was done in thick walled heavy black glass bottles from the same soda fountain equipment. This was done at the same time as the customers were being served, and was sold back to the same fountain customers to take back home with them (see Joseph Hawkins ads from the *Baltimore Whig* of July 1810).

These heavy thick walled bottles were used for much the same reason stoneware bottles were used in England - they could more safely absorb mishandling and the variable pressures of the primitive mineral water manufacturing equipment that existed before 1817.

In England bottling was primarily done in heavy stoneware bottles. The English use of stoneware bottles rather than light weight glass egg bottles had little to do with the so-called English glass tax

(1745-1845) or the medicine (soda water) tax (1804-1833), as many other historians have claimed. It was because of the continual danger of serious explosions. Other researchers simply failed to discover and properly understand the dangerous and primitive nature of the bottling equipment in highly pressurized manufacturing operations.

Newly discovered historical and archaeological evidence is conclusive.
The metallic materials of that time simply lacked the physical properties to contain the variable pressures even if an adequate engineering design had been found (in the period 1790-1820). *(See archaeological examples of these early valves on the next few pages.)* So either the vessels being filled or the equipment itself exploded causing death or serious injury.

Thus, either ceramic or heavy black glass bottles had to be used, and in England the heavy black glass bottles were taxed, so ceramic was cheaper even if the product lost its carbonation and became flat due to the porosity of the ceramic bottles. As was mentioned earlier, the earliest Schweppes invoices offering glass egg bottles as an option to their normal stoneware bottles, are dated 1821. This was likely because the use of light weight egg bottles was nearly impossible in England as well as the United States until James S Ewing's equipment was invented and patented in 1817.

The first adequate engineering design was not patented in England but in the United States in 1817. Not until 1817 was a remote controlled pressure throw valve developed and patented by James S. Ewing (hydrant valve). James S. Ewing improved his mineral water manufacturing equipment in 1823 evidenced by his second patent and the Magellanic Premium Award of 1823.

This technology was also applied to city water systems (hydrants), house plumbing systems (freeze valves), mineral water equipment, and tavern equipment used to dispense porter, ale, and cider. This equipment was far superior to any other known at that time, including all known patented English, U.S., or Irish mineral water bottling equipment.

Another serious problem was corrosion. James S. Ewing claimed to have largely eliminated this by using lead in his mineral water manufacturing equipment. Of course the underlying health issue was not recognized at that time and one can only wonder if slow poisoning was preferable to being exposed to an explosion?

(See:

- *William Hamilton 1809 patent # 3232 - equipment to prepare soda water,*
  & 1814 patent # 3819 - carbonating and filling equipment,
- *Joseph Bramah (passed away 1814) and William Russell (Bramah's understudy)*
  - equipment to manufacture soda water (1820),
- *David Grant patent # 3805 - pump to draw off soda water,*
- *Nicolas Paul - report to National Institute of France December 1799 & repeated in London 1802,*
- *Joseph Hawkins 1809 US patent - soda fountain improvements and inventions,*
- *inter alia.)*

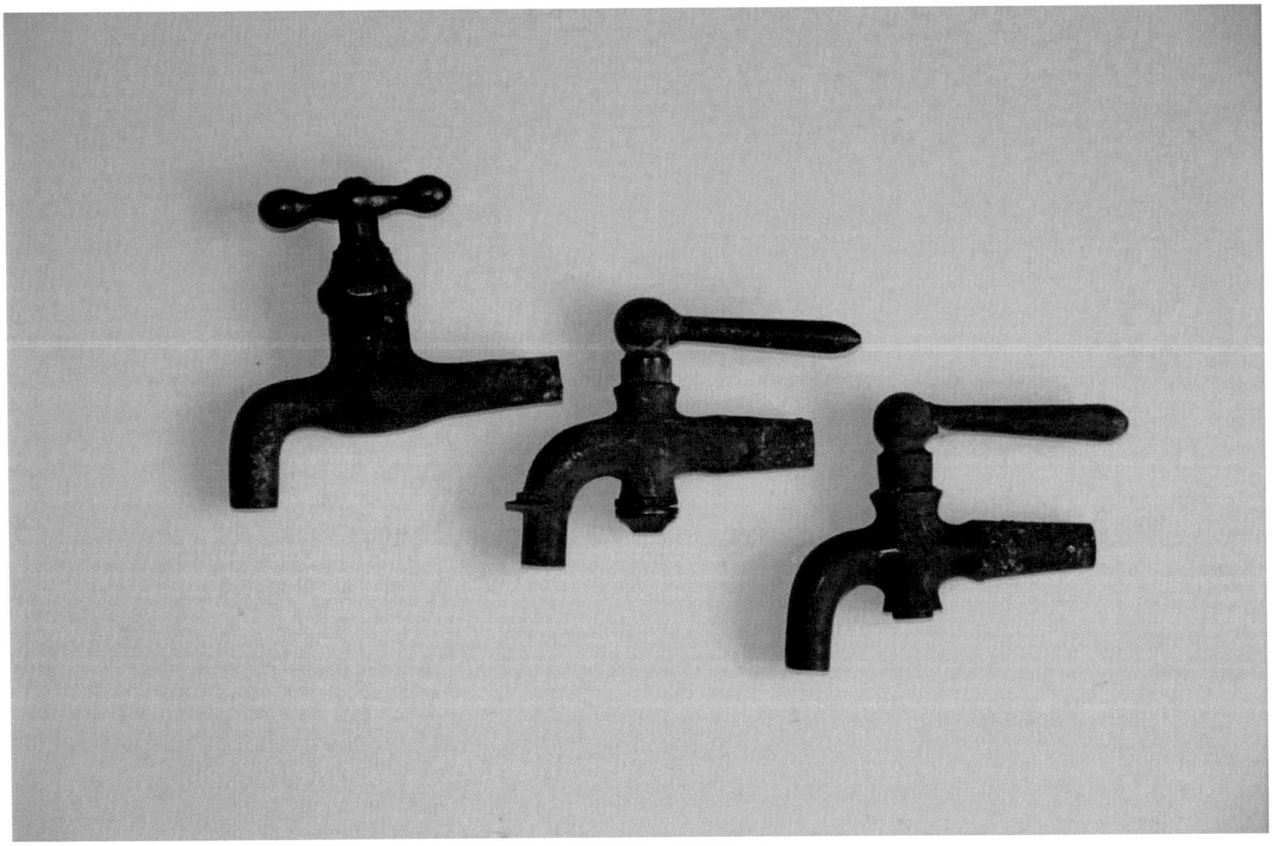

Pictured are a series of embossed water valves from the early to mid 1800's showing the transition from a primitive tapered valve into the more modern form. The suspected dating is confirmed by archaeological context and dated historical records verifying the embossed names on each valve. The earliest are taper shaft valves (in the center and lower right) – these are from 1830 - 1840. In the late 1840's this design evolved into the safer, less leaky, and more precise water valve shown in the upper left (1850 – 1860). All are made of brass metal of imprecise strength due to impurities. They are pictured in the condition recovered - none have been restored or altered. By the 1850's Ewing's lever valves proved far easier to use in automated manufacturing operations and they replaced the twist and taper shaft valves pictured above.

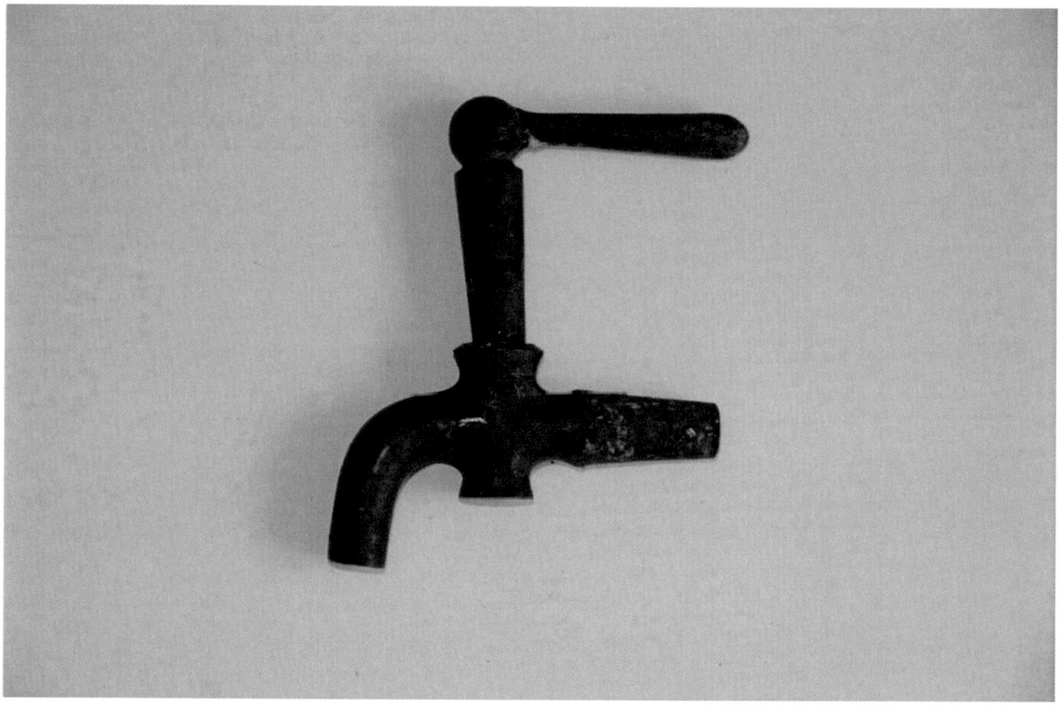

Pictured is a "*taper shaft*" valve from the 1830's very similar to the primitive valves shown in mineral water manufacturing / fountain equipment patent drawings (1790-1820). Although the faucet part was modified for loading bottles, it made little difference. "*Taper shaft*" brass valves were leaky and prone to explosion under high pressure. Nor could they precisely regulate the pressure of the mineral water being loaded. Thus the bottles frequently exploded as well.

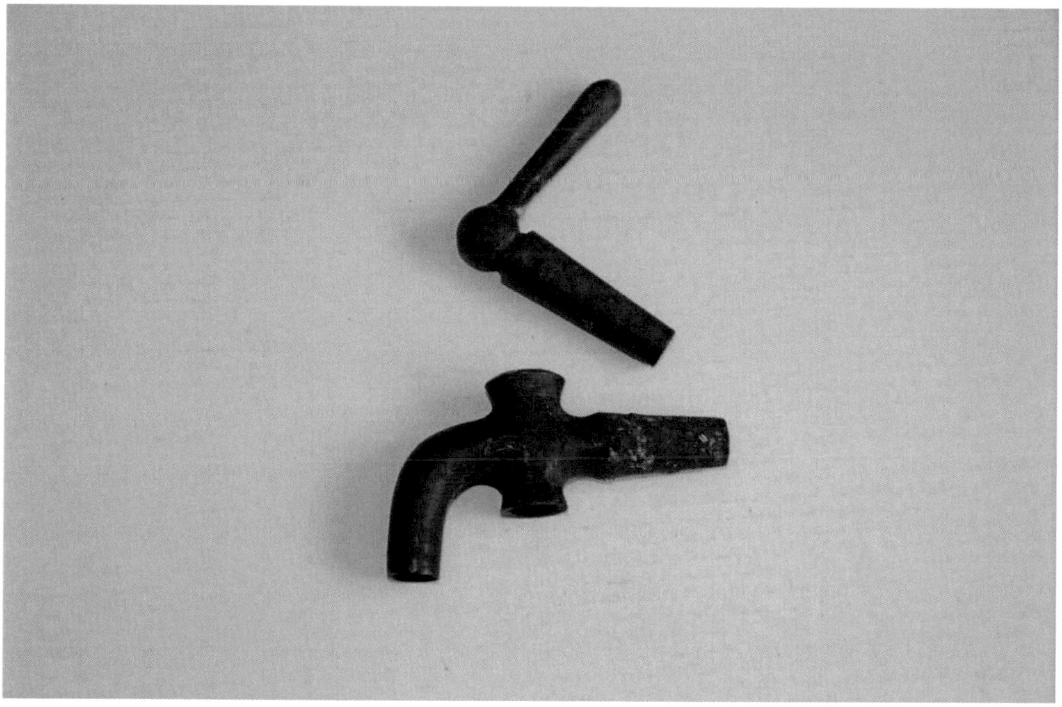

APPENDIX D

Cullen Bottle Recovery Area - Wood & Ridge Road

This is a partial list of Philadelphia directory entries showing commercial and hotel activity at one site in the area. One hotel proprietor from the 1840's, "*Henry G. Douglass*", yielded his own marked artifacts. He continued until 1848. No embossed "*Douglass, Hoffman, or Wellbank*" artifacts were found in the 1850's through 1870's artifact layers. The table below shows *H.G. Douglass* was a proprietor at this location from approximately 1842 through 1848. In 1849 *H.G. Douglass* is listed in Philadelphia directories as a "*Bottler*" located in West Philadelphia. *Henry C. Blumner* from the late 1820's and early 1830's later became a famous engine manufacturer in Philadelphia. It is interesting to note that he started out as a baker before making this transition. It illustrates that social evolution involving significant career change has occurred for hundreds of years and that human yearning occurs throughout the generations. It is not just confined to our current time period and life ways.

Year	Listed Name	Philadelphia Address	Occupation	Ref
1816				
1817				
1818				
1819				
1820				
1821				
1822				
1823				
1824				
1825	Rhoades, Charles	18 Ridge Road	Cake Baker	37
1828				
1829	Blummer, Henry C.	18 Ridge Road	Baker	2
1830	Blumner, Henry C.	18 Ridge Road	Baker	2
1831	Blumner, Henry C.	18 Ridge Road	Baker	2
1833	Blumner, Henry C.	18 Ridge Road	Baker	2
1835	Brannan, J.	NW c. Wood & Ridge Rd.	Tavern Keeper	2
1837				1
1839				1
1840	Moore, Alexander	Cor. Ridge Road & Wood	Oyster House	1
1841	Moore, Alexander	Cor. Ridge Road & Wood	Oyster House	1
1842				1
1843	Douglass, Henry	Ridge Road & Wood St.	?	1
1844	Douglass, Henry G.	Ridge Road & Wood St.	?	1
1845	Douglass, Henry G.	Ridge Road & Wood St.	?	1
1846	Douglass, Henry G.	Ridge Road & Wood St.	Tavern	1
1847	Douglass, Henry G.	Ridge Road & Wood St.	?	1
1848	Douglass, Henry G.	Ridge Road & Wood St.	?	1
1849	Hoffman, D.E.	Ridge Road & Wood St.	Tavern	1

1850	Hoffman, D.E.	Ridge Road & Wood St.	Tavern	1
1851	Hoffman, D.E.	Ridge Road & Wood St.	Tavern	1
1852	(not listed)			1
1853	Wellbank, Henry	18 Ridge Road	Tavern	1
1854	(not listed)			1
1855	Wellbank, Henry	18 Ridge Av.	Hotel	1
1856	Wellbank, Henry	18 Ridge Av.	Hotel	1
1857	Wellbank, Henry	18 Ridge Av.	Hotel	1
1858	(not listed)			1
1859	Wellbank, Henry	916 Ridge Av.	Hotel	1
1859	Wellbank, Henry	914 Ridge Av.	Porter House	B5
1860	Wellbank, Henry	Philadelphia, 13th Ward	Hotel Keyser	192
1860	Wellbank, Henry	914 Ridge Av.	Tavern	1
1861	Wellbank, Henry	914Ridge Av.	Tavern	1
1862	Wellbank, Henry	914 Ridge Av.	Tavern	1
1863	Wellbank, Henry	914 Ridge Av.	Tavern	1
1864	Wellbank, Harry	914 Ridge Av.	Hotel	1
1870	Wellbank, Henry	914Ridge Av.	Liquors	95
1875	(not listed)			95

The "*Henry G. Douglass*" artifacts discovered were not previously known in Philadelphia and are of "*first impression*" here. Pictures of these "*Union Glass Works*" embossed porter bottle shards, with archaeological context circa. 1844–1848, are shown in the following two pages.

The bottle is embossed, "*H. G. Douglass / N.W. Cor. / Ridge Road / & Wood St.*" The reverse side is "*Union Glass Works / Philada*" in one mold variant. In another mold variant the words Porter / Ale / Cider are embossed as well as a very large font size for the glassworks embossing. The color is medium cobalt blue typical of "*Union Glass Works*" bottles from the mid to late 1840's (such as the script *Heiss* bottles etc.).

It should be noted the "*Douglass*" directory entries correlate well with the "*Union Glass Works*" period of activity as well as with other known marked artifacts from that glassworks. The majority of marked "*Union Glass Works*" artifacts date from the late 1840's. Two different mold styles were recovered although both were somewhat similar. These artifacts are undisputable facts in support of our theory of the area's significant "*Hotel–Tavern*" use over a wide spectrum of time (1800 – 1890).

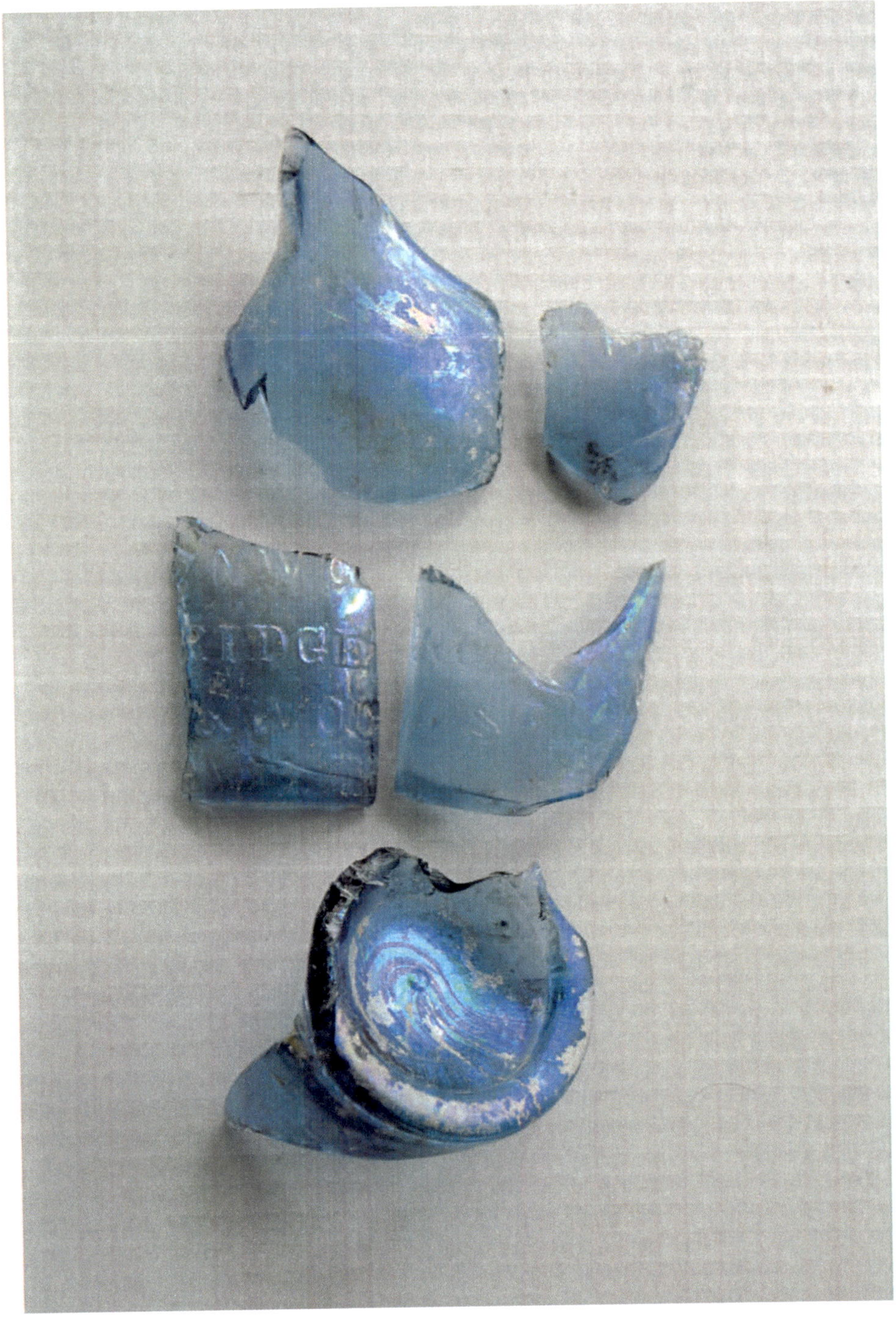

"H.G.Douglass" porter bottle shards are shown above – this artifact was not previously known by the amateur or professional archaeological community in and around the Philadelphia region, (*mold variant 1*).

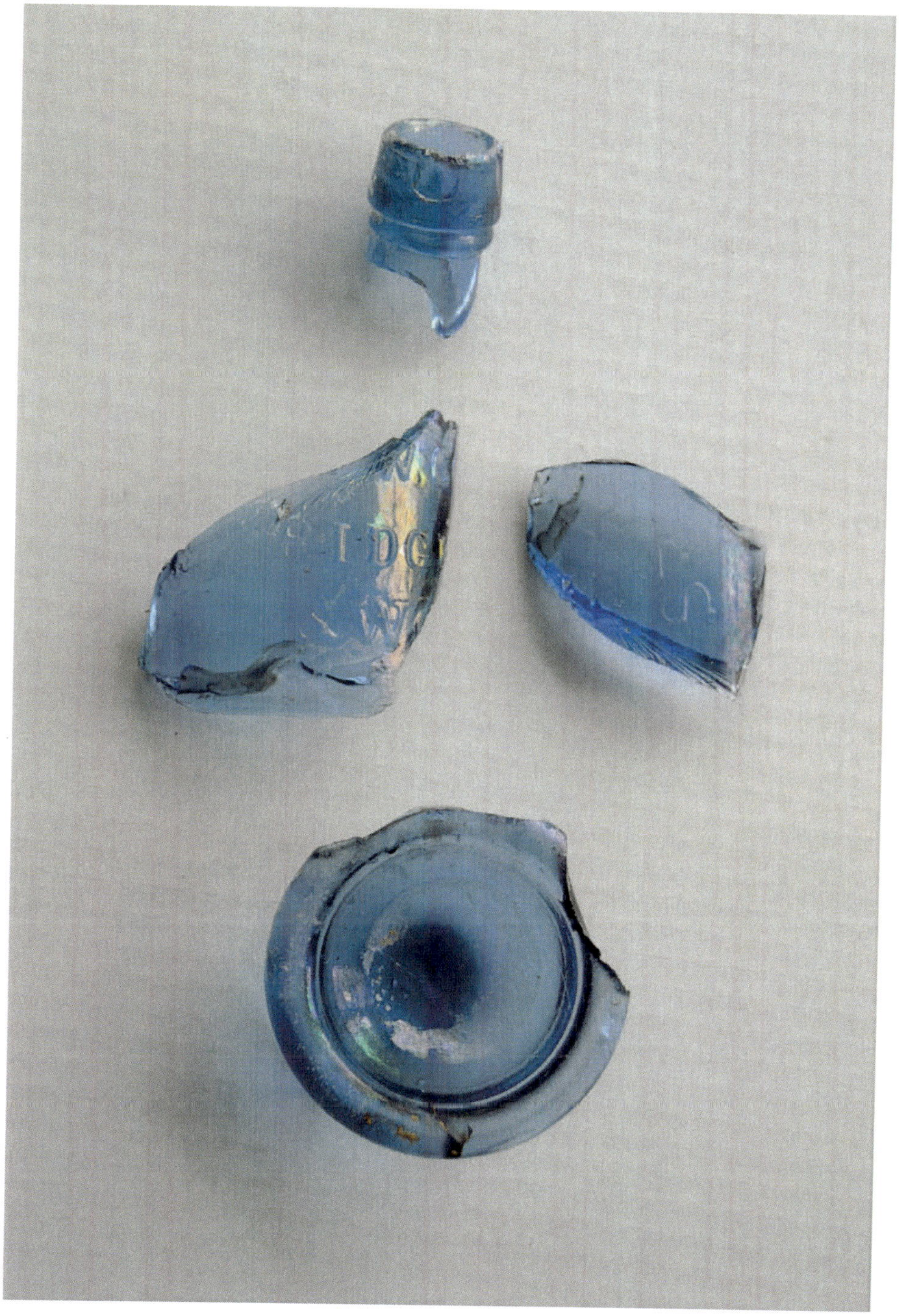

"H.G.Douglass" porter bottle shards are shown above from "*mold variant 2*" - *(large glassworks font size as well as "Porter/Ale/Cider" style embossing)*.

APPENDIX E

Chronology of "*Wood Street & Ridge Road*" Changes

The early history of this area reveals a terminus. Wood Street originally terminated at Ridge Road near the corner of 9th and Vine Streets (1802 – 1817). It is interesting to note Ridge Road was described as Roads, (plural), from 1802-1810. Ridge Road and Wissahiccon Road actually were two roads combined into one. Each began life separately and ultimately ran together over time as population burdens increased and the roads expanded. It appears Ridge Road was the original city name. Then later it was referred to by its country name, "Wissahiccon Road" for several decades. Then back to the city name, "Ridge Road", by 1840. This road eventually carried a traveler to the Wissahiccon creek area, northwest of Philadelphia, near where it meets the Schuylkill River.

Ridge Road (Wissahiccon Road) was one of many toll roads in Philadelphia. It had a number of toll gates - each gate manned by a collector. For instance, in *Whitely's 1820 Philadelphia Directory & Register, John French*" is listed as "*Toll Gatherer at the 1st gate on Ridge Road*". The toll collectors usually lived near the gates as a necessity of the job. Other significant toll roads around Philadelphia included Frankford Road, Germantown Road, and Lancaster Turnpike. Often in times of public disorder the rates charged would fluctuate widely. Thomas Jefferson claimed he paid more than $80 after the yellow fever panic of 1793 to travel from Baltimore to Germantown (northwestern Philadelphia).

The table on the next page illustrates how the "*Wood and Ridge Road*" area changed over time. During these early years it was a good area for a tavern, restaurant, or hotel. Since four major streets were in close proximity and two terminated into the others, (*Wood St., Ridge Road, 9th Street, and Vine Street*), it would seem to be a natural location for travelers to rest and enjoy a healthy mineral water to settle their stomachs and disposition.

Around 1817 and 1818, Wood Street was expanded westward to the Schuylkill River. Previously Wood Street dead ended into Ridge Road, (Wissahiccon Road). This further increased the building and activity in the area. **Thereby "food, *hotel, tavern*" combinations likely thrived. The archaeological evidence I recovered on site, confirmed this. In summary, the area of "*Wood and Ridge*" was used by "food, *hotel, tavern*" combinations from around 1800 through 1890.**

When Wood Street was expanded westward across Ridge Road around 1818, it happened to correspond to the same year John Cullen was selling (egg bottled) mineral waters. Whether this means anything can be debated but it is another unusual coincidence in the life of John Cullen that culminated with your author, 187 years later, re-discovering this great American.

Year	Street Name	Directions each street travels in.
1799	(not listed)	
1800	(not listed)	
1801	(not listed)	
1802	Wood Street	York to Ridge Roads bet. Vine & Callowhill
1803	Wood Street	York to Ridge Roads bet. Vine & Callowhill

1804	Wood Street	York to Ridge Roads bet. Vine & Callowhill
1805	Wood Street	York to Ridge Roads bet. Vine & Callowhill
1806	Wood Street	York to Ridge Roads bet. Vine & Callowhill
1807	Wood Street	York to Ridge Roads bet. Vine & Callowhill
1808	Wood Street	York to Ridge Roads bet. Vine & Callowhill
1809	Wood Street	York to Ridge Roads bet. Vine & Callowhill
1810	Wood Street	York to Ridge Roads bet. Vine & Callowhill
1811	Wissahiccon Road (Ridge Road)	NW from corner of N 9th & Vine Sts.
	Wood Street (N.L.)	from 190 N 2nd to Wissahiccon Road
1813	Wissahiccon Road (Ridge Road)	NW from corner of N 9th & Vine Sts.
	Wood Street (N.L.)	from 190 N 2nd to Wissahiccon Road
1814	Wissahiccon Road (Ridge Road)	NW from corner of N 9th & Vine Sts.
	Wood Street (N.L.)	from 190 N 2nd to Wissahiccon Road
1816	Wissahiccon Road (Ridge Road)	NW from corner of N 9th & Vine Sts.
	Wood Street (N.L.)	from 190 N 2nd to Wissahiccon Road
1817	Wissahiccon Road (Ridge Road)	NW from corner of N 9th & Vine Sts.
	Wood Street (N.L.)	from 190 N 2nd to Wissahiccon Road
1818	Wissahiccon Road (Ridge Road)	NW from corner of N 9th & Vine Sts.
	Wood Street (N.L.)	from 190 N 2nd to Schuykill River
1819	Wissahiccon Road (Ridge Road)	NW from corner of N 9th & Vine Sts.
	Wood Street (N.L.)	from 190 N 2nd to Schuykill River
1820	Wissahiccon Road (Ridge Road)	NW from corner of N 9th & Vine Sts.
	Wood Street	from 190 N 2nd to Schuykill River
1825	Wissahiccon Road (Ridge Road)	NW from corner of N 9th & Vine Sts.
	Wood Street	from 190 N 2nd to Schuykill River
1830	Wissahiccon Road (Ridge Road)	NW from corner of N 9th & Vine Sts.
	Wood Street	from 190 N 2nd to Schuykill River
1835	Wissahiccon Road (Ridge Road)	NW from corner of N 9th & Vine Sts.
	Wood Street	from 190 N 2nd to Schuykill River
1840	Ridge Road	NW from corner of Vine & N 9th Sts.
	Wood Street (N.L.& S.G)	from 2nd to Schuykill bet. Vine & Callowhill

These entries are taken from the "*street lists*" in Philadelphia directories for the years indicated.

APPENDIX F

Acknowledgments

As with any endeavor of this type, I have received help and encouragement from so many. This acknowledgment seems inadequate to convey my full appreciation and respect to those listed below, as well as to those whom I may have mistakenly omitted.

First and foremost are my digging partners who over a lifetime of discovery have shared a joint passion for archaeological discovery. They have given of their time and money - and that which cannot be purchased at any price – their friendship. With deep respect, thank you, Ernie and Steve for 35 years of wonderful adventures. To those who first illuminated my passionate journey, thank you Winnie and others. To those who shared and supported me in these adventures, thank you Dove, Fred, Eve, Don Z., Don D., Doug, Sam, Evan and so many others.

Often without knowing me personally, the following have trusted me, allowed me into their homes and institutions, and offered their genuine friendship and help. Thank you...

Nancy R. Miller – *University of Pennsylvania* Archives and Records Center, Philadelphia, Pa.
Dr. Eric L. Schmetterling - Collector
Ernie Strong
Sam Devoe
Evan Devoe
Andrew Bain - Thompkins McCaw Library, *Virginia Commonwealth University,* Richmond Va.
Jolene Milot – James Branch Cabell Library, *Virginia Commonwealth University,* Richmond Va.
Charlene Peacock - *The Library Company of Philadelphia,* Philadelphia, Pa.
Linda Wisniewski - *The Library Company of Philadelphia,* Philadelphia, Pa.
Phillip Lapsansky - *The Library Company of Philadelphia,* Philadelphia, Pa.
Cornelia S. King - *The Library Company of Philadelphia,* Philadelphia, Pa.
Roy Goodman - *American Philosophical Society*, Philadelphia, Pa.
Valerie Lutz - *American Philosophical Society*, Philadelphia, Pa.
Richard Boardman - *Free Library of Philadelphia,* Philadelphia, Pa.
David T. Baugh - *City of Philadelphia, Department of Records, City Archives,* Philadelphia, Pa.
Doug Shutler
Don Dzuro
Jim Hagenbuch
Robert Maglies
Greg Gifford
Jim Hall – Collector
John Odell – Historian & Researcher
Canady Library - *Bryn Mawr College*, Philadelphia, Pa.
Olga Tsapina – Curator, American Historical Manuscripts, *Huntington Library,* San Marino, Ca.
Alan Jutzi – Curator rare books, *Huntington Library,* San Marino, Ca.
Alex Peck – *Antiques Scientifica*, Charleston, Illinois
Ruth Nyblood – *U.S. Patent Office*, Washington, D.C.

Bibliography

OSD – Original Source Documents

American Philosophical Society, Magellanic Premium Award – February 20, 1823 Recipient James S Ewing, APS Archives III, 1 – 2 items Box 3 – includes engineering diagrams of his some of his inventions. Location: American Philosophical Society, Philadelphia, Pa.

"An Essay on Naturalization and Allegiance…" Author: John F. DuMoulin, Published by Daniel Rapine, Washington City, 1816, John Cullen written repeatedly on the front endpaper, Location: Huntington Library, San Marino, Ca. Rare Books, Call No: 190835

"Atlantic Journal of Medicine", entitled "Sketch of the Life of Dr. John Cullen." Atlantic Journal of Medicine, v.1, no. 3 (October 1883), pages 191-199) by Dr. T. Pollard. Location: Thompkins McCaw Library, Virginia Commonwealth University, Richmond Va.

Aurora General Advertiser", published daily for William Duane 110 & 112 Walnut St., Philadelphia Pa. - daily newspaper. Locations: The Library Company of Philadelphia, Pa., and private collections.

"Baltimore Whig", printed & published by B. Irvine, cor. of Gay & Water Streets, Baltimore Maryland - daily newspaper. Locations: Maryland State Archives, Baltimore, Md., The Library Company of Philadelphia, Pa., and private collections.

Charlotte Howard Cullen Letters to Samuel Taylor of December 9, 10, 1844, concerning marital troubles with Dr. John Cullen, 1844-1846. Location: Brock Collection, Huntington Library, San Marino, Ca. (No call numbers).

Hexamer & Locher pre-Civil War multi-volume Philadelphia map series (approximately 1859). Location: Free Library of Philadelphia, 1901 Vine Street, Philadelphia, Pa.

John Cullen handwritten Letter – December 28, 1818; Subject was a request to University Of Pennsylvania Medical School for credit towards his Medical Degree. Granted by Dr. John Redman Coxe and majority of staff. Location: University of Pennsylvania, University Archives & Records Center, Philadelphia, Pa.

John Cullen Alumni records – Location: University of Pennsylvania, University Archives & Records Center, Philadelphia, Pa.

John Cullen handwritten medical bill dated 1824, Richmond Va. With full signature – 34. Courtesy Alex Peck – "Antiques Scientifica", Charleston, Illinois. Location: private collection.

Philadelphia Mayor's Court, Naturalization records, October 28, 1817, Microfilm Roll # 21.17 (1814-1838), Docket 130.3 – 7 vols., as well as original docket page. Location: City of Philadelphia, Department of Records, City Archives, 3101 Market St. Philadelphia, Pa. 19104.

REF – Reference Documents

Arch Otolaryngol Head Neck Surgery Vol. 126 No. 3, March 2000 (*2000;126:353-359*) - The Cervical Wound of General James Longstreet .

"The Evolution of Glass Bottles for Carbonated Drinks", by Olive Talbot, - "Post Medieval Archaeology" Vol. 8, 1974;

OSD – Original Source Documents
(continued)

Philadelphia Directory entries – Various Years, 1799 through 1880. (i.e. Whitley's, DeSilver's, McElroy's, etc.), Locations: Free Library of Philadelphia, 1901 Vine Street, Philadelphia, Pa., The Library Company of Philadelphia, Pa., Canady Library - Bryn Mawr College, Philadelphia, Pa., University of Pennsylvania Library, Philadelphia, Pa. and private collections.

Philadelphia Medical Museum 1809 – Editor, John Redman Coxe, annual journal (book publication) 1805 – 1811. Locations: American Philosophical Society, Philadelphia, Pa. and The Library Company of Philadelphia, Pa.

"The Union, United States Gazette and True American", published by Bronson and Smith, 67 Dock St. corner Bank St., Philadelphia Pa. - daily newspaper. Locations: The Library Company of Philadelphia, Pa. and private collections.

United States original X Patent Indexes – Washington, D.C., 1790 – 1829. Indexes of all known patents granted by "U States letters Patent" for the years indicated. Location: US Patent Office, Washington, DC.

Index

A

B

C

D

E

G

H

J

L

M

N

P

R

S

T

U

V

W